*Selected Methods of Clinical Chemistry
Volume 11*

Selected Methods of Emergency Toxicology

Contributors to This Volume

Submitters

Keith Adams • Roy E. Altman, Jr. • Roger L. Boeckx • Charles A. Bradley • Larry A. Broussard • Robert W. Dalrymple • Linda D. Dorie • Christopher S. Frings • Richard H. Gadsden, Sr. • Victoria R. Giblin • E. Philip Halpern • Horace E. Hamilton • Stephen A. Hite • Walter I. Hofman • Earle W. Holmes • Gerald Long • John A. Lott • James E. Love, Jr. • Jerry L. McHan • Alexandros A. Pappas • William H. Porter • Francis Avery Ragan, Jr. • C. Ray Ratliff • Mona Beckman Royder • Philip W. Rutter • Frank M. Stearns • Ernest W. Street • Donald E. Sutherland • E. Howard Taylor • C. Steven Terry

Evaluators

Eleanor Berman • Kenneth E. Blick • Larry A. Broussard • Yale H. Caplan • R. T. Chamberlain • Gerald E. Clement • H. Patrick Covault • Karl M. Doetsch • Stephen W. Duckett • Ted W. Fendley • William D. Hemphill • David C. Hohnadel • Catherine H. Ketchum • Joseph E. Manno • Stan Marenberg • John T. McCall • F. Leland McClure • Richard E. Mullins • Linda Pellegrino • Gaylon A. Peyton • William H. Porter • Cecelia H. Queen • Francis A. Ragan, Jr. • C. Ray Ratliff • C. Andrew Robinson, Jr. • T. Sabapathy • Lynne Selby • Gary L. Smith • Steven J. Steindel • E. Howard Taylor • Bernard C. Thompson • Richard T. Tulley • Ann Warner • John Wojcieszyn

Selected Methods of Clinical Chemistry, Volume 11

Selected Methods of Emergency Toxicology

Editor-in-Chief
Christopher S. Frings
Senior Vice-President, Technical Services
Director, Clinical Chemistry and Toxicology
Medical Laboratory Associates
Birmingham, AL 35256

Co-Editor
Willard R. Faulkner
Professor of Biochemistry Emeritus
Vanderbilt University Medical Center
Nashville, TN 37212

Series Editor
Virginia S. Marcum

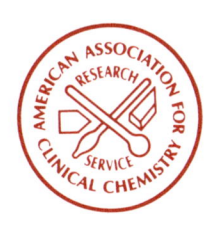

AACC PRESS
American Association for Clinical Chemistry
1725 K Street, N.W.
Washington, DC 20006

1986

BOARD OF EDITORS
Selected Methods of Clinical Chemistry

Willard R. Faulkner, Editor-in-Chief, Department of Biochemistry, Vanderbilt University Medical Center, Nashville, TN 37212

Paige K. Besch, Department of Obstetrics and Gynecology, Baylor College of Medicine, Houston, TX 77030

Peggy R. Borum, Institute of Food and Agricultural Sciences, University of Florida, Gainesville, FL 32611

Charles A. Bradley, Clinical Chemistry, Vanderbilt University Medical Center, Nashville, TN 37232

Martin Fleisher, Biochemistry Department, Memorial Sloan-Kettering Cancer Center, New York, NY 10021

Donald T. Forman, Clinical Chemistry Laboratories, The North Carolina Memorial Hospital, Chapel Hill, NC 27514

Christopher S. Frings, Clinical Chemistry and Toxicology, Medical Laboratory Associates, Birmingham, AL 35256

Richard H. Gadsden, Sr., Clinical Laboratories, Medical University of South Carolina, Charleston, SC 29425

Phillip J. Garry, Clinical Nutrition Laboratory, University of New Mexico, Albuquerque, NM 87131

Judith A. Hopkins, Corporate Technology Sourcing, Travenol Laboratories, Inc., Round Lake, IL 60073

John A. Lott, Department of Pathology, The Ohio State University, Columbus, OH 43210

Samuel Meites, Clinical Chemistry, Children's Hospital, Columbus, OH 43205

George E. Nichoalds, 5956-F Shadetree Lane, Raleigh, NC 27612

Herbert K. Naito, Division of Laboratory Medicine and Division of Research, The Cleveland Clinic Foundation, Cleveland, OH 44106

Henry C. Nipper, Clinical Chemistry, Beth Israel Hospital, Boston, MA 02215

Thomas C. Stewart, Medical Laboratory of Baton Rouge, Baton Rouge, LA 70806

Library of Congress Catalog Card No. 53-7099
ISBN 0-915274-31-0

© 1986, by the American Association for Clinical Chemistry, Inc. All rights reserved. No part of this book may be reproduced or transmitted, or translated into a machine language without written permission from the publishers.

Printed in the United States of America.

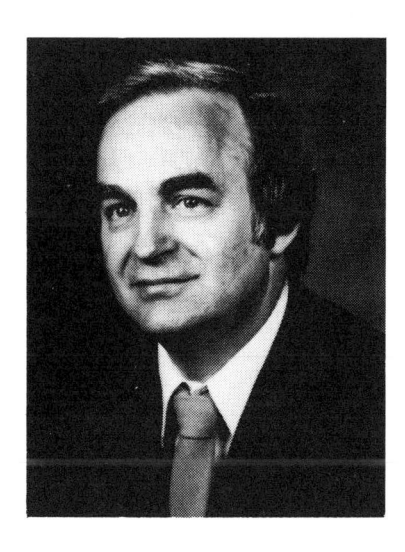

Harry L. Pardue

From time to time, a "non" clinical chemist enters the field and makes such marked contributions as to stand out prominently among his clinical chemistry colleagues. Such a man is Harry L. Pardue, an analytical chemist with initial scientific interests far removed from the field of clinical chemistry as it was known two decades ago. He earned B.S. and M.S. degrees in chemistry at Marshall University, Huntington, WV, in 1956 and 1957, respectively, and a Ph.D degree in analytical chemistry from the University of Illinois in 1961. At that time, he joined the faculty of the Department of Chemistry at Purdue University, advancing to Professor in 1969; currently he is head of that department. Dr. Pardue had developed an active, sustained interest in the application of electronics to analytical chemical problems. This interest was expressed through the development of novel methods and instruments for kinetic measurements and computations, spectroscopic detection systems, and automation of analyses. He was among those who noted the advantageous features of fast kinetic analyses during the early 1970s when this technique was being developed. More recently, he has exploited the capabilities of imaging sensors and array detectors in the development of analytical systems based on data obtained from the rapid scanning of spectra.

Dr. Pardue has served on the editorial boards of *Analytical Chemistry* and *Clinical Chemistry*. At present he is the American editor for *Analytica Chimica Acta*. He has also been active as a member of the AACC Standards Committee, and of the Analytical Chemistry Division's Advisory Committee, Oak Ridge National Laboratory.

Over the course of his career, Dr. Pardue has published more than a hundred papers describing his research in the area of clinical and bioanalytical chemistry.

During the last two decades he has directed a doctoral program; many of his students are now leaders in clinical chemistry, analytical chemistry, and toxicology.

Recognition for his work has been expressed through the following awards:

ISCO Award for significant contributions to biochemical instrumentation, 1978.

Boehringer Mannheim Award for outstanding contributions to clinical chemistry in a specific area, 1978.

Samuel Natelson Award of the Fisher Scientific Co. for originality, initiative, and contributions to the advancement of clinical chemistry, 1982.

In 1980 his alma mater, Marshall University, honored him as their distinguished alumnus of the year.

Beyond his work as an analytical clinical chemist, Harry Pardue is a leader who continually provides an uncommon stimulus to his colleagues and to his students. For this and numerous other contributions, we proudly dedicate this volume to him.

The Editors

Foreword

During the last several decades, investigators working in numerous laboratories around the world have provided the means to a better understanding of toxic substances, including their chemical reactions in and their pharmacologic effects on the host. Within this same time, chemists, engineers, and scientists in other disciplines have developed instruments and techniques for detecting and quantifying a wide variety of toxicants. Rigid standards and ways of assuring the quality of analytical results have not been neglected, because in emergency clinical settings there would not be time to correct errors and because the ever-present specter of legal complications requires documented evidence of analytical accuracy. Thus, all of the needed resources are, theoretically, at hand for the laboratorian to aid the clinician in diagnosing and treating a patient who is in a critically toxic state. Although there are literally hundreds of toxic agents, only a few are commonly encountered in emergency situations. It is these few that cause most of the trouble and that are the focus of this book.

The authors have brought together in this special volume much of the knowledge and expertise on emergency analytical toxicology that has been gathered over the years through basic and applied research. They have written the chapters in such a manner as to carry this important information out of the purely theoretical realm and into the eminently practical.

The information presented should be a valuable resource in educational projects and classroom work as well as in the analytical laboratory. The increasing interest in emergency toxicology in countries undergoing industrialization gives this book widespread international usefulness.

The analytical needs of emergency toxicology constantly challenge the clinical chemist to apply advances in related potentially useful methodologies. This book primarily presents current applications of rapid procedures involving spectrophotometry, chromatography, and atomic absorption spectrometry. The procedures provide a sound base that can in the future be extended through applications of advances in isolation and concentration techniques, immunochemistry, radioreceptor assays, inductively coupled argon plasma spectroscopy, and computer data-handling systems. Such methods have the potential to provide more rapid qualitative analysis of unknown specimens and more specific quantitative analysis for specific analytes in emergency toxicology.

Gerald R. Cooper

Past President, AACC, and
Research Medical Officer
Clinical Chemistry Division
Center for Environmental Health
Centers for Disease Control
Public Health Service
U.S. Department of Health and
  Human Services
Atlanta, GA 30333

Preface

Many clinical laboratories are confronted with a relatively new responsibility, namely, offering toxicological determinations. To do this properly, laboratories must have reliable and accurate procedures with which to respond to the diverse demands currently being placed on them.

The Editor-in-Chief of this volume has received frequent requests over the years for advice in choosing a suitable method for determining a particular toxic substance. In most instances a specific method could be recommended to solve the problem at hand. Given this experience and background, we concluded that a collection of time-tested procedures was needed to help laboratories cope with the problems of emergency toxicology.

The production of the volume has adhered closely to the basic tenets established during the last three decades for books in the *Selected Method* series:

• Each chapter is written by a chemist, toxicologist, or physician thoroughly familiar with the procedure through its use in his or her own laboratory.

• To ensure that all methods would work in any laboratories in which they were properly used, the methods have been evaluated by one or two additional scientists, working independently of the author and of each other. This evaluation is practical—not an "armchair" review. Although time-consuming and sometimes difficult, the actual setting up and trying of a method by analysts other than the author is a special and invaluable feature that sets *Selected Methods* apart from most other texts. It is a virtual guarantee that the method will do what it is purported to do. For two chapters labeled "provisional," we were unable to set up this evaluation step; however, the procedures have been used in the Submitters' laboratories and not only are clinically useful, but also have been the standard of quality for many years.

• All methods have been chosen with a concern for relative simplicity and rapid turnaround time, consistent with reliability and accuracy.

This volume is not all-inclusive; it was not meant to be. Our intention was to include procedures for only those toxic agents most likely to be encountered in a hospital setting. Of course, there is not complete agreement among toxicologists and physicians as to just which procedures should be placed in an "emergency" category: we recognize and respect these differences of opinion.

Throughout the process of selecting what methods to include, we have wanted to present procedures that would allow laboratory scientists to prepare their own reagents. Thus we have avoided commercial kits, which often contain "secret" (proprietary) ingredients and are likely to be modified from time to time by the manufacturer.

We acknowledge the indispensible role played by the AACC publications board in launching this volume. Also, we would have has a much slower start without the assistance and support of Scott Hunt in the AACC national office. We are especially grateful to Virginia S. Marcum for the care and astuteness she applied in editing each chapter. Finally, we express our appreciation to all Submitters and Evaluators for giving their time and expertise. They were the actual builders of this volume. We hope their efforts will prove worthwhile.

Christopher S. Frings
Editor-in-Chief

Willard R. Faulkner
Co-Editor

CONTENTS

Dedication: Harry L. Pardue v

Foreword, *Gerald R. Cooper* vii

Preface viii

THE HANDLING OF TOXICOLOGY SPECIMENS ... 1
Submitters: Walter I. Hofman and E. Philip Halpern
Evaluators: Yale H. Caplan, Eleanor Berman, and R. T. Chamberlain

QUALITY ASSURANCE IN TOXICOLOGY 5
Submitter: Roy E. Altman, Jr.
Evaluator: Bernard C. Thompson

SCREENING PROCEDURES
I. Multiple Drugs by Thin-Layer Chromatography . 13
Submitter: Larry A. Broussard
Evaluators: Ted W. Fendley and Linda Pellegrino

II. Multiple Drugs by Gas-Liquid Chromatography . 22
Submitters: Francis Avery Ragan, Jr., Stephen A. Hite, and Victoria R. Giblin
Evaluator: William D. Hemphill

III. Basic Drugs in Urine 26
Submitters: Robert W. Dalrymple and Frank M. Stearns
Evaluator: Gerald E. Clement

IV. Phenothiazines 30
Submitter: Christopher S. Frings
Evaluators: C. Ray Ratliff and Ann Warner

V. Chlorinated Hydrocarbons 31
Submitters: Francis Avery Ragan, Jr., and Victoria R. Giblin
Evaluators: Joseph E. Manno and William D. Hemphill

ACETAMINOPHEN BY LIQUID CHROMATOGRAPHY 33
Submitters: William H. Porter, Linda D. Dorie, and Philip W. Rutter
Evaluators: Stephen W. Duckett, David C. Hohnadel, and E. Howard Taylor

ACETAMINOPHEN BY COLORIMETRY 37
Submitters: Frank M. Stearns and Robert W. Dalrymple
Evaluator: Larry A. Broussard

ALCOHOLS IN BIOLOGICAL FLUIDS BY GAS CHROMATOGRAPHY (AUTOMATED HEAD-SPACE METHOD) 40
Submitters: Richard H. Gadsden, Sr., and C. Steven Terry
Evaluator: Bernard C. Thompson

ARSENIC BY SPECTROPHOTOMETRY (PROVISIONAL) 44
Submitter: C. Ray Ratliff

BARBITURATES BY SPECTROPHOTOMETRY 47
Submitters: James E. Love, Jr., and John A. Lott
Evaluators: Larry A. Broussard and Lynne Selby

BROMIDE IN SERUM BY SPECTROPHOTOMETRY 51
Submitter: Charles A. Bradley
Evaluator: Kenneth E. Blick

CARBOXYHEMOGLOBIN BY SPECTROPHOTOMETRY 53
Submitter: Earle W. Holmes
Evaluators: H. Patrick Covault and T. Sabapathy

CYANIDE AND THIOCYANATE BY MICRODIFFUSION AND SPECTROPHOTOMETRY . 57
Submitters: Horace E. Hamilton, Ernest W. Street, Mona Beckman Royder, and Keith Adams
Evaluators: F. Leland McClure and Gaylon A. Peyton

ETHANOL IN BIOLOGICAL FLUIDS BY ENZYMIC ANALYSIS 63
Submitters: Richard H. Gadsden, Sr., and E. Howard Taylor
Evaluators: Steven J. Steindel, Francis A. Ragan, Jr., and Karl M. Doetsch

ETHCHLORVYNOL BY SPECTROPHOTOMETRY .. 66
Submitter: Christopher S. Frings
Evaluators: Cecelia H. Queen and C. Ray Ratliff

ETHYLENE GLYCOL BY GAS-LIQUID CHROMATOGRAPHY 69
Submitters: William H. Porter and Linda D. Dorie
Evaluators: C. Andrew Robinson, Jr., Catherine H. Ketchum, and E. Howard Taylor

IRON IN SERUM BY SPECTROPHOTOMETRY 72
Submitter: Charles A. Bradley
Evaluator: Kenneth E. Blick

LEAD IN WHOLE BLOOD BY FLAMELESS ATOMIC ABSORPTION SPECTROPHOTOMETRY 75
Submitter: Roger L. Boeckx
Evaluator: John T. McCall

MERCURY IN URINE BY ATOMIC ABSORPTION SPECTROPHOTOMETRY, WITH USE OF A MERCURY HYDRIDE SYSTEM 79
Submitter: Jerry L. McHan
Evaluator: Gary L. Smith

METHAQUALONE BY SPECTROPHOTOMETRY .. 82
Submitter: Larry A. Broussard
Evaluators: Richard T. Tulley, C. Andrew Robinson, Jr., and Catherine H. Ketchum

OSMOLALITY OF SERUM FOR EVALUATING THE ACUTELY INTOXICATED PATIENT 85
Submitters: Alexandros A. Pappas and Richard H. Gadsden, Sr.
Evaluators: William H. Porter and Richard E. Mullins

SALICYLATE BY SPECTROPHOTOMETRY 89
  Submitters: Donald E. Sutherland and John A. Lott
  Evaluator: Stan Marenberg

TRICYCLIC ANTIDEPRESSANTS BY GAS-LIQUID CHROMATOGRAPHY WITH A NITROGEN-SENSITIVE DETECTOR (PROVISIONAL) 93
  Submitters: Jerry L. McHan and Gerald Long

TRICYCLIC AND TETRACYCLIC ANTIDEPRESSANTS BY LIQUID CHROMATOGRAPHY 96
  Submitters: E. Howard Taylor and Richard H. Gadsden, Sr.
  Evaluator: John Wojcieszyn

Index 101

Selected Methods of
Emergency Toxicology

The Handling of Toxicology Specimens

Submitters: Walter I. Hofman, *Department of Laboratory Medicine, Roxborough Memorial Hospital, Philadelphia, PA, 19128; Department of Pathology, Temple University School of Medicine, Philadelphia, PA; Office of the Gloucester County Medical Examiner, Woodbury, NJ*

E. Philip Halpern, *Department of Laboratory Medicine, Memorial Hospital, Roxborough, Philadelphia, PA, and E. P. Halpern Consulting Associates, Philadelphia, PA*

Evaluators: Yale H. Caplan, *Chief Toxicologist, Office of the Chief Medical Examiner, Baltimore, MD 21201*

Eleanor Berman, *Chief Toxicologist, Division of Biochemistry, Cook County Hospital, Chicago, IL 60612*

R. T. Chamberlain, *Clinical Chemistry, Toxicology, Verterans Administration Medical Center, Memphis, TN 38104*

Introduction

The vast majority of requests for toxicology are handled as emergency specimens by most clinical laboratories. Not infrequently, however, days, weeks, or months after the analyses are complete, the laboratory is informed that the specimen may have "medical-legal" consequences.

Laboratories in general have established procedures for maintaining patient and specimen identification for both emergency and routine testing. The legal description for this procedure is "maintaining the integrity of the specimen" (Chain of Custody/Evidence). The proper specimen(s) must be collected, properly preserved, and properly related to pertinent clinical-historical information (1,2). Then, adequate toxicologic testing can be requested and meaningful results (either positive or negative) obtained. The most common breakdowns in laboratory procedures occur before and during the collection of the specimen and in identifying the specimen before analysis (3).

Informed Patient Consent

Frequently, specimens for emergency toxicological analyses are from patients who are unconscious, unresponsive, or in an altered state of awareness. Voluntary consent for treatment or for collection and testing of specimens cannot be obtained from these patients. Nonetheless, whenever possible, written permission should be obtained.

Analytical Result (Evidence)

The results of body fluid testing may be considered "evidence." Examples of evidence are blood samples for determining if the patient was impaired, unfit, or intoxicated by alcohol while operating a motor vehicle, or urine samples for determining whether morphine or its derivatives were present in a suspected drug addict (4,5).

Maintaining the Integrity of the Specimen (Chain of Custody/Evidence)

The following is the optimal system (3) for maintaining the integrity of the specimen. Each laboratory may wish to modify these procedures somewhat, but essentially the following information should be recorded:

1. Who obtained the specimen (e.g., venipuncture), where and when, using which antiseptic.
2. Which tests were requested for the specimen, by which physicians, for what purpose.
3. Who transported the specimen to the laboratory.
4. Who received and who accessioned the specimen.
5. Who processed and who analyzed the specimen.
6. Who checked the validity of the results and who reported them.

Many of these items are self-explanatory and are part of the required documentation of the laboratory request slips. Although not necessary in routine situations, a record should be kept of how much of the specimen was used in obvious medical-legal situations. Laboratories accredited by either the College of American Pathologists (CAP), the Joint Commission for the Accreditation of Hospitals (JCAH), or the Centers for Disease Control (CDC) must retain a copy of the analyses for at least two years. Most (more than 75%) medical-legal inquiries arise within the first two years after the analysis. Many institutions have a method of restrictive access to toxicology specimens with suspected medical-legal implications. The information needed to maintain the integrity of the specimen can be noted on the back of the laboratory report copy. We maintain lists of names, signatures, and initials of past and current laboratory personnel.

Collection of Specimens

Table 1 lists the specimens that should be obtained and retained for general and specific analyses. The availability of sophisticated methodologies means that most toxicological testing can be performed on the universal specimen, blood (4,6). Other body fluids (e.g., urine or gastric contents) are desired to confirm or further identify trace quantities of a substance originally found in blood (2,7).

Table 1. Collection of Body Fluids for Toxicological Examinations

Source	Tube type	Requirements	Type of study
Routine analyses			
Blood			
Serum	Red top	Two 10-mL or one 15-mL	
Plasma	Green or lavender top (heparin or EDTA)	Two EDTA tubes or one 10-mL heparinized tube	Methodology dependent: 1. It is recommended that heparinized tubes *not* be used for hypnotics and tranquilizers. 2. Samples for psychoactive drugs, such as imipramine, should be submitted *frozen*, if they cannot be processed in-house.
Whole	Gray or lavender top (fluoride/oxalate or EDTA)	Two 7-mL tubes	Carbon monoxide, alkyl nitrite, lead and cyanide, volatiles.
Urine	Container with plastic lid	At least 50 mL	Drugs and drug metabolites, including drugs of abuse, volatiles.
Gastric contents	Container with plastic lid	At least 50 mL (1st aspirate plus 1st washing)	Orally ingested intoxicants.
Alternative analyses			
Saliva	Container with plastic lid	Two 5-mL	Cannabinoids, volatiles, including alcohol, benzodiazepines, etc.
Cerebrospinal fluid	Plastic spinal tray tubes	All available are suitable	Volatiles, drugs, etc. when blood sample is limited or unavailable.

Urine is a particularly useful and economical specimen for excluding or detecting a broad range of drugs, intoxicants, and poisons (7). Notable exceptions are carbon monoxide, alkyl nitrite, lead, and cyanide, for which whole blood is essential.

Precautions in Specimen Collection

1. Many times, initial clinical information may be incorrect or incomplete. Whenever possible, blood, urine, and gastric contents should be submitted to the laboratory (7-9). The type of specimen the laboratory will analyze will be influenced by any specific drug requested and the clinical information provided.

2. The venipuncture site should be cleansed with a nonalcohol (e.g., Betadine®), or noniodine (e.g., Zephiran®) preparation (10). This precludes potentially significant contamination in collection and analysis and eliminates controversy in judicial proceedings.

3. For ethanol analysis, the blood-collection tube should remain stoppered at all times to minimize any potential loss of volatile compounds. Where possible, a separate sample should be obtained for the analysis of volatiles. If this is not practical, then testing for alcohols and other volatiles should be undertaken first, before testing for other analytes.

4. A urine specimen should be submitted concurrently with the blood specimen. It may be necessary to catheterize the patient (4).

5. Laboratories involved in collecting specimens for drug abuse, rehabilitation, or probation testing must ensure positive patient identification by monitoring specimen collection.

6. Stomach contents should be obtained either by inducing vomiting (e.g., with syrup of ipecac) or by gastric intubation. If intubation is used, collect both the first aspiration and the first washing with 100 mL of isotonic saline (NaCl 9 g/L) in separate, properly labeled containers, and keep the specimen(s) cold during transport to the laboratory.

7. The laboratory should be supplied with a list of known medications that the patient currently has access to (prescribed or otherwise) and, if available, should be given samples of the medications themselves (Figure 1) (11). Laboratories that regularly analyze medication intoxications should have available the FDA National Drug Code Directory (Govt. Printing Office, Washington, DC) and annual Red/Blue Books (American Druggist, Hearst Corp., New York, NY), which detail medications not shown in the *Physician's Desk Reference (PDR)* (12). The Pharmaceutical Manufacturers Association guide

PATIENT _____
AGE _____ SEX _____
DOCTOR _____
DATE _____

1. Complete this requisition form, including patient symptoms/signs.
2. Submit stamped/patient data miscellaneous laboratory slip.
3. Submit 30 mL urine, 5 mL serum (one red-top tube) and, if available, 10 mL of the initial gastric aspirate or vomitus.

PATIENT CURRENT MEDICATION _____

DRUGS SUSPECTED _____

ESTIMATED TIME OF INGESTION _____

DRUGS ADMINISTERED PRIOR TO
SPECIMEN COLLECTION _____

SPECIMEN SUBMITTED	COLLECTED BY	TIME
☐ BLOOD SERUM		
☐ URINE		
RANDOM/24 HOURS		
☐ GASTRIC CONTENT		
☐ OTHER SPECIFY _____		

TIME STAMP

PATIENT SYMPTOMS/SIGNS:

GENERAL:
_____ CHILLS
_____ CONGESTED CONJUNCTIVAE
_____ DEHYDRATION
_____ DIZZINESS
_____ FEVER
_____ FLUSHING
_____ HEADACHES
_____ HYPERTENSION
_____ HYPOTENSION
_____ HYPOTHERMIA
_____ NASAL CONGESTIONS

_____ NAUSEA
_____ SWEATING

CARDIOVASCULAR
_____ ARRHYTHMIAS
_____ CYANOSIS
_____ TACHYCARDIA

GI:
_____ BLOOD LOSS
_____ DIARRHEA
_____ VOMITING

CNS:
_____ AGITATED
_____ ATAXIA
_____ COMATOSE
_____ CONVULSION
_____ DISORIENTATION
_____ HALLUCINATION
_____ HYPERTENSION
_____ LETHARGY
_____ MUSCLE TWITCHING
_____ NYSTAGMUS
_____ HYPERVENTILATION

_____ PUPILS CONSTRICTED
_____ PUPILS DILATED
_____ HYPERSALIVATION
_____ SPEECH SLURRED
_____ STUPOR
_____ TREMORS
_____ URINARY RETENTION
_____ VISION BLURRED
_____ VIOLENT
OTHERS, SPECIFY: _____

SPECIMEN	TEST RESULTS

TIME STAMP

RESULT CALLED TO _____ BY _____ TIME _____

NOTES
1. <u>Screening results should be considered presumptive and not for forensic use.</u>
2. Unless reported present, the following drugs and/or metabolites were screened for, but not detected:
Serum—Barbiturates (amobarbital, butabarbital, pentobarbital, phenobarbital, secobarbital); Benzodiazepines (chlordiazepoxide, clonazepam, diazepam, flurazepam, lorazepam, oxazepam, prazepam); Ethanol; Phencyclidine (PCP); Phenytoin; Salicylates.
Urine-Acetaminophen; Amphetamines (amphetamine, metamphetamine); Antidepressants (amitriptyline, nortriptyline, imipramine, desipramine, doxepin); Antihistamines (dimenhydrinate, diphenhydramine); Carbamazepine; Ephedrine; Ethchlorvynol; Flurazepam; Meprobamate, Methaqualone; Narcotics (codeine, morphine, methadone, meperidine, propoxyphene);-Phenothiazines; Phencyclidine (PCP).
Gastric Content—All drugs listed under serum and urine.

Fig. 1. Request form for drug screen

describes medications on the basis of symbols and shapes not related to the manufacturer's abbreviations or code-detailed in the *PDR*.

8. In general, despite use of multiple drugs and attendance by multiple physicians, patients rarely utilize more than one pharmacy to obtain their medications. Thus unmarked or generic pills, capsules, and fluids can usually be identified with the cooperation of the pharmacy involved. A telephone call to the pharmacy can save a lot of valuable time and prevent a diagnostic or therapeutic misadventure.

9. Gastric contents or emesis are most useful in determining whether an acute drug ingestion has occurred, as in a suicidal intoxication. The presence of significant amounts of drug(s) is probably important and may explain the clinical situation (13). The converse, however, does not hold true. The findings of nondetectable to trace amounts of a substance is not conclusive because gastric contents empty into the small bowel in 2 to 4 h or less. Finally, the amount of substance present has no relationship to the degree of intoxication, which depends on the amount of drug or metabolite present in the target organ(s) or bloodstream.

10. When an inadequate specimen has been submitted, the toxicology laboratory can often obtain material for examination from that which was submitted for routine chemistry, hematology, or microbiology analysis. Usually the lavender hematology (EDTA) or blue coagulation (citrate) tubes as well as cerebrospinal fluid specimens are stoppered, refrigerated, and preserved.

11. The laboratory should make use of forensic/toxicological expertise, which is readily available in all metropolitan areas. The forensic pathologists and toxicologists, usually associated with a medical examiner/coroner's office, are more than willing to share their knowledge. They are usually familiar with the problem and can offer specialized advice on specimen choice and other matters. Over the past 15 years we have found that, in life-threatening situations, they are always available to perform an esoteric toxicology analysis, even at 02:00 h.

Preservation of Specimens

1. Specimens should be refrigerated as soon as possible after collection to minimize bacteriologic action (i.e., alcohol production, etc.) (14). Most drugs in whole-blood samples do not deteriorate while refrigerated.

2. Specimens to be frozen should be transferred into freezer-proof plastic vials and sealed with a plastic cap. Do *not* use cellophane-type tape to seal vials.

3. Refrigerated storage space in laboratories being at a premium, laboratories should consider keeping frozen aliquots. Five hundred 1.8-mL vials containing frozen aliquots can be stored in four 23 × 23 cm racks, which for the average 100- to 200-bed hospital would constitute one to two years' worth of specimens. This procedure is already followed by many hospital transfusion services, which retain aliquots of pretransfusion sera on all transfused patients.

4. Certain test-tube stoppers may cause interference with certain analytes. The plasticizer tributoxyethyl phosphate (TBEP), for example, although no longer used as commonly as several years ago, interferes in the analysis of methyprylon and thallates (15). Stoppers lubricated with silicone have also been reported to cause interferences.

Other Body Fluids with Potential for Future Toxicological Applications

Saliva, which can be obtained noninvasively, is likely to play an increasingly important role in the detection of all types of drugs (5,16). If both saliva and limited blood samples are available, saliva can be used for qualitative analyses of drugs, blood for quantifying the drugs detected in the saliva. Saliva/plasma ratios for many drugs have been published (9), and newer, more sensitive, methodologies are being developed to determine even lower concentrations of drugs in saliva.

Cerebrospinal fluid is not routinely used in emergency toxicological situations. However, there are clinical situations where the diagnosis of drug intoxication is not initially suspected. Cerebrospinal fluid obtained for neurological evaluation may provide the only clue to the origin of the clinical problem, when blood and urine collected at the time of admission are no longer available.

In conclusion, stringent specimen collection protocols must be followed. The collection of adequate specimens and pertinent clinical information is of paramount importance. Frozen aliquots of samples should be retained for possible further analyses.

The Submitters thank Dr. Frederic Rieders, Forensic Toxicologist, Willow Grove, PA, for his assistance and critical comments.

References

1. Blanke RV. Analysis of drugs and toxic substances. In *Fundamentals of Clinical Chemistry*, NW Tietz, Ed., WB Saunders Co., Philadelphia, PA, 1976, pp 1100-1103.
2. DiMaio VJM. Trace evidence and the pathologist. In *Clinics in Laboratory Medicine*, VJM DiMaio, Ed., WB Saunders Co., Philadelphia, PA, 1983, pp 355-365.
3. Wilber CG. Legal considerations for the clinical chemist. *Am Clin Prod Rev* 2(6), 20-28 (1983).
4. Kaye S. The collection and handling of the blood alcohol specimen. *Am J Clin Pathol* 74, 743-746 (1980).
5. Peel HW, Perrigo BJ, Mikhael NZ. Detection of drugs in saliva of impaired drivers. *J Forens Sci* 29, 185-189 (1984).
6. Garriott JC. Interpretive toxicology. *Op. cit.* (ref. 2), pp 367-385.
7. Garriott JC. Toxicology—choice of specimens, drug distribution and metabolism. *Forens Sci Gaz* 2(3), 1-3 (1971).
8. Curry A. *Poison Detection in Human Organs*, 2nd ed., CC Thomas Co., Springfield, IL, 1969, pp 5-23.
9. Kaye S. *Handbook of Emergency Toxicology*, 3rd ed., CC Thomas Co., Springfield, IL, 1970, pp 21-108.
10. Dubowski KM, Essary NA. Contamination of blood specimens for alcohol analysis during collection. *Abst Rev Alcohol Driving* 4(2), 3-8 (April-June, 1983).
11. Hepler BR, Sutheimer CA, Sunshine A. The role of the toxicology laboratory in emergency medicine. *J Toxicol Clin Toxicol* 19, 353-365 (1982).
12. *Physicians' Desk Reference*, 38th ed., Medical Economics Co., Oradell, NJ, 1984.
13. Garriott JC. Choice of specimens for toxicologic testing. *Forens Sci Gaz* 6(2), 4-6 (1975).
14. Garriott JC, Hatchett D, Dempsey J. Stability of drugs in autopsy blood. *Forens Sci Gaz* 8(4), 1-3 (1977).
15. Perel JM, Stiler RC. Effect of specimen collection on the analysis of haloperidol, a neuroleptic drug. *Clin Chem* 27, 1102 (1981). Abstract.
16. Idowu OR, Caddy B. A review of the use of saliva in the forensic detection of drugs and other chemicals. *J Forens Sci Soc* 22, 123-135 (1981).

Quality Assurance in Toxicology

Submitter: Roy E. Altman, Jr., *Department of Pathology, Clinical Chemistry and Toxicology, Medical College of Georgia, Augusta, GA 30912*

Evaluator: Bernard C. Thompson, *Toxicology Department, SmithKline Bioscience Laboratories, Inc., King of Prussia, PA 19406*

Introduction

Results produced in a toxicology laboratory can have profound effects on the lives of the individuals being tested. In many industries today, employees who operate vehicles or other dangerous equipment and thus need to be free from the influence of drugs are screened for drugs in their urine—both current and potential employees. For these and other reasons, hospitals and private and referral laboratories are performing more and more toxicology assays each year. Accurate and precise results are important because any false-negative or false-positive responses could result in termination of employment, imprisonment, improper medical treatment, or treatment with incompatible drugs.

Although toxicology predates the field of clinical chemistry by many years, it has been the clinical chemists who have led many toxicologists into effective quality-assurance programs, primarily because of the different volumes of data in the two fields. It is easier to see the need for quality control in serum glucose results, for example, which may involve hundreds of analyses daily, than in analyses of biological samples for ethchlorvynol, which a toxicologist may see only a few times a month. This low-volume situation has lulled many toxicologists into exempting themselves from quality-assurance programs, for reasons of economics, unstable analytes, and the small number of samples for a single procedure. Many workers fail to realize the need to include quality-control samples when a standard curve is run each assay day. With the widespread use of therapeutic drug monitoring (TDM), however, many toxicologists now realize the need for an in-depth quality-assurance program.

Quality assurance may be defined as a system involved in monitoring all aspects of data production, beginning with collecting samples, developing methods, preparing quality-control material, conducting surveys, monitoring results, and reporting results. Thus quality-assurance programs are even more difficult to establish in hospital toxicology laboratories than in reference laboratories. Many suppliers of diagnostic products have addressed the need for control serum for TDM and, indeed, have essentially solved this problem for laboratorians who use immunoassays. However, these control sera contain many drug analytes and are not useful for chromatographic or spectrophotometric methods. For those procedures the drugs must be carefully chosen to eliminate interference. Many companies marketing multicomponent controls offer a computer service as part of the "package," to make the daily handling of data less time consuming. Currently, a few urine-matrix products are becoming available that can be useful for quality assurance when screening urine for drugs of abuse by thin-layer chromatography (TLC).

Toxicologists in reference laboratories have long been accustomed to making their own quality-control samples because of the lack of products that fit their scheme of analysis. These individuals have solved their quality-control problems the difficult way, by trial and error. In this chapter I will describe methods that may be useful to institutions starting or expanding their toxicology service and will discuss pitfalls in quality-assurance programs that plague most of us. Below are definitions of some terms pertinent to this chapter:

Accuracy—agreement between the best analytical estimate and its true value

Blank—sample that closely matches the matrix of the analytical specimen without the presence of the analyte being analyzed

Blind specimen—sample submitted under an assumed name, the expected value and the identity of which are unknown to the analyst

Coefficient of variation (CV)—relative standard deviation; the standard deviations (s) expressed as a percentage of the mean ($\bar{x}$) (*1*): CV = ($s/\bar{x}$) × 100%

Detection limit—the smallest quantity of analyte that can be measured with a reasonable amount of confidence

Interfering substance—any substance that mimics the analytical behavior of an analyte in question or otherwise prevents its accurate determination

Matrix—material used to dissolve or dilute the analyte

Precision—agreement of results from one determination to another

Proficiency test specimen—a sample of known value but submitted to the laboratory as an unknown test specimen

Quality-control program—a program for the study of those errors that are the responsibility of the laboratory, and the procedures used to recognize and minimize them; all errors arising within the laboratory between the receipt of the specimen to the dispatch of the report are included (*2*)

Quality-control specimen—a sample of known expected value, analyzed through the same procedure as a patient's sample

Specificity—the degree of accuracy with which a technique can measure a single analyte in the presence of other analytes

Split sample—a sample that has been divided into at least two parts and submitted for analysis separately to the same or different laboratories

Standard—a sample of known concentration used to prepare calibration curves from which analytes in patients' and quality-control specimens are measured

Unknown specimen—a sample for which the expected value is not known by the person performing the analysis

Materials and Methods

Analytical Standards

All toxicologists share the frustration of trying to procure pure samples of analytes and their metabolites. For some analytes a Drug Enforcement Agency (DEA) license is required, although some chromatographic supply houses offer a few high-purity control substances dissolved in methanol that do not require a DEA license to purchase or use. Pure drug materials should be stored in a securely locked cabinet, and a record of material received and used should be kept and inventoried every two years. Evans (3) reviewed these regulations in 1972.

Any laboratorian serious about developing toxicology procedures and a toxicology quality-assurance program should have at least the following two catalogs: Alltech-Applied Science, State College, PA, and U.S. Pharmacopoeial Reference Standards, Rockville, MD. Together, these two sources can provide most of the analytical standards needed in a quality-assurance program. Several other sources that should not be overlooked are: various pharmaceutical houses (addresses listed in *Physicians' Desk Reference*, Medical Economics Co., Oradell, NJ); reagent suppliers, e.g., Sigma Chemical Co., St. Louis, MO; and chromatographic supply houses, e.g., Supelco, Inc., Bellefonte, PA, and Pierce Chemical Co., Rockford, IL.

Although many of the standards obtained through the sources listed are of high quality and may have the purity indicated on the label, one should verify the actual purity by analysis in the laboratory. The record of purity for a standard thus not only verifies the manufacturer's claims but also can serve as a baseline if later verification is needed. Ultraviolet absorptivity characteristics of a substance are commonly used to verify its purity. For example, according to the *Merck Index* (10th ed.; Merck & Co., Inc., Rahway, NJ, 1983, p 1042), phenobarbital dissolved in pH 10 buffer has an absorbance at 240 nm of 431 for a 10 g/L solution in a 1-cm cell. If no absorptivity data can be obtained or if additional verification is needed, one should consider using mass spectrometry, gas chromatography, and (or) liquid chromatography to detect impurities.

Finally, the local pharmacy is a ready source of drug materials, although it may be necessary to separate fillers and binders from drugs obtained in this manner, which may thus require extraction. One must also identify the salt moiety of the analyte in question.

Stock and Working Standards

The *Merck Index* is a valuable aid in determining solubility of standards in various solvents, e.g., water, ethanol, or methanol. For those analytes not listed, simple trial and error may be required to determine solubility. An ultrasonic bath can help dissolve standards in solvents. The analytical balance used should be accurate within 0.1 mg because most analytes used in these analytical procedures require microgram quantities of pure drug to be measured.

Concentrations of analytes are expressed in terms of their free form, not the salt. Thus, to obtain a 1.0-mg sample of chlordiazepoxide, one should weigh 1.12 mg of chlordiazepoxide hydrochloride (336.21/299.75 = 1.12). Allowance for the salt form is especially troublesome in drugs obtained from a pharmacy. Propoxyphene, for example, is marketed both as the hydrochloride and the napsylate salt. Water of hydration and water as a contaminant must also be dealt with by calculation or by properly drying the standard before weighing. Usual concentrations of stock standards range from 0.5 to 2 g/L. Label these for concentration, drug lot number, solvent used, date prepared, and an appropriate expiration date and store at −10 °C.

Finally, standards are diluted with a biological matrix, divided into aliquots, and frozen (−15 to −20 °C) for use later. These solutions should also be labeled for lot number, date prepared, and expiration date.

Internal Standards

When methods of analysis are chosen, the use of internal standards cannot be overemphasized. Using these as monitoring devices will improve quality-assurance program performance. Everyone is aware of the value and uses of internal standards when performing gas and liquid-chromatographic analyses; few, however, recognize their importance in TLC. Introduction of internal standards in TLC procedures will monitor extraction, chromatography, and staining procedures. Choosing internal standards with extraction and chromatographic properties similar to those of the analytes in question is very important. Johnson and Stevenson (4) list six criteria an internal standard should meet.

Note: Evaluator B.C.T. noted also the importance of internal standards in improving reproducibility and monitoring various procedure parameters.

Design of Quality-Control Material

Vendors of quality-control material, in an effort to design marketable material, have added as many as 33 analytes to a single serum control (Table 1). Some of these

Table 1. Drugs Included in TDM Controls

acetaminophen	desipramine	lithium	propranolol
N-acetylprocain-amide	digoxin	methotrexate	quinidine
	disopyramide	netilmicin	salicylate
amikacin	ethosuximide	nortriptyline	streptomycin
amitriptyline	gentamicin	phenobarbital	theophylline
carbamazepine	imipramine	phenytoin	tobramycin
chloramphenicol	kanamycin	primidone	valproic acid
clonazepam	lidocaine	procainamide	vancomycin

products are usable for immunoassays and do indeed elucidate the specificity of these assays. Of course, no matter how many analytes are added, there always seems to be one left out or several included at the "wrong" concentration. The package inserts from these products provide valuable information about stability, compatibility, specificity, and the concentration of analytes to be considered when designing one's own quality-control material. Table 1 lists some drugs that could be included in a TDM control for immunoassay.

Although immunoassays available in kits are methods of choice for many analytes, several analyses are not available in kit form. For these the toxicologist must use chromatography or spectrophotometry, methodologies for which commercial products containing large numbers of analytes are not useful; for these, toxicologists must design their own quality-control material.

First, analytes and the concentration to be added to each control material lot should be selected with care. For example, if the analysis involves gas chromatography, one should select analytes that do not co-elute or have excessively close retention times. Injection of each separate working standard solution used in preparing quality-control material not only identifies the retention time of the standard, but also rules out the possibility of interfering peaks in the final solution that may have originated from starting material. Second, the concentrations of analytes used should reflect clinically relevant situations rather than concentrations at either extreme of the assay range of linearity. Third, analytes should be chosen that have similar extraction characteristics, as determined by recovery studies during development of the method. Thoma (5) recommends putting a single acid analyte in a control material used for monitoring bases: if everything is operating properly, the acid analyte will not be seen during the analysis; if the acid is detected, one should suspect problems with the procedure.

Quality-Control Serum

Although salvaged plasma may not be recommended (6) for use as a matrix for control material, it is frequently the only choice, if one cannot obtain drug-free serum collected in glass. Lipemic, hemolyzed, and icteric pools should be avoided; hospital laboratory serum is often positive for hepatitis HB_sAg and cannot be used. However, some procedures can help make salvaged plasma useful as a matrix for preparing quality-control samples. If serum is needed, the procedure described by Proksch and Bonderman (7) in 1976 is recommended. If plasma is desired, the abundance of caffeine and over-the-counter drugs makes it necessary to clean up most of the pooled plasma to be used for toxicology. This can be done effectively as follows:

1. Add activated charcoal (Sigma, no. C4386), 4 g/L, and let stand with occasional mixing for 1 h.
2. Freeze, then let thaw at room temperature.
3. Centrifuge, then repeat steps 1 and 2.
4. Repeat step 2 once more.
5. Filter through an 0.2-μm pore-size filter to remove any bacteria, which might later cause analyte loss (8).
6. Add 1 g of sodium azide preservative per liter. [Omit step 6 for a matrix pool to be used in procedures that require a ferric ion, e.g., the widely used method of Trinder for salicylate. A chromogen formed from sodium azide and ferric ion interferes with these assays (9). Adding a preservative can also be avoided if the quality-control material will be used up or discarded within one day after thawing (or within three days if stored refrigerated between use).]

This drug-free pool is then tested through every procedure that will be used for analyzing the patients' and quality-control specimens. Aliquots of this material are stored frozen and labeled as blank specimens for use later.

The pool can now be used to prepare quality-control material by adding the appropriate working standard solutions. For standards dissolved in ethanol or methanol, be careful not to exceed a 30 mL/L proportion of alcohol as the standards are being added (5). Either use sufficiently concentrated standard solutions or evaporate some of the alcohol from the standard solution before adding the matrix material. If evaporation is used—especially if heat is applied—be careful not to lose any other volatile components that may have been added. If results from analyzing a sample of this batch are acceptable, put aliquots into screw-top tubes labeled with lot number and expiration dates (one year for most analytes), then freeze the material (-15 to -20 °C). Glass containers are not acceptable; use plastic to avoid breakage during freezing. Polypropylene leakproof mailing vials from W. Sarstedt Inc., Princeton, NJ, or from Evergreen Scientific, Los Angeles, CA, are recommended.

If calibration standards and quality-control material are prepared from the same lot number of pure standard, the analyst should be aware of the critical need to verify the purity of this standard.

Quality-Control Urine Samples

Obtaining drug-free urine does not present any unusual problems, but some precautions should be taken. After collection, the urine should be frozen at the end of each day without added preservative. Common over-the-counter medications (e.g., aspirin, antihistamines, and cold preparations) are sometimes taken by donors who forget or don't consider that these are drugs. Make separate collections for nonsmokers and smokers, because nicotine and its metabolites are present in urines from the latter.

Thaw the total volume needed, removing the insoluble salts by gravity filtration through a porous filter paper, then refilter through an 0.2-μm pore-size filter to remove any bacteria (8).

Analyze the filtered urine by each procedure to be used for the patients' samples. After blank aliquots are stored frozen in screw-top plastic vials, prepare the final product by adding the analytes. Again, be careful not to add excessive amounts of alcohol in this step. The amount of alcohol that can be tolerated can be easily determined by taking a patient's urine that contains the drug in question and re-analyzing this sample with various amounts of alcohol added. Through careful record keeping, this information can be accumulated for most common analytes. Label the prepared quality-control material with a lot number, the date prepared, and an expiration date (one year for most analytes) and store it in a freezer, not a frost-free model, at -15 to -20 °C.

Verification of Quality-Control and Calibration Material

Standard reference materials for drugs in a biological matrix are not readily available commercially at this time except for two multi-component anticonvulsant products available through the National Bureau of Standards, Washington, DC. One of these sera contains phenytoin, ethosuximide, phenobarbital, and primidone; the other, valproic acid and carbamazepine. Therefore, laboratorians must either resort to calibration standards and quality-control materials intended for use with immunoassay kits or prepare their own.

Assume that calibration standards and quality-control material have just been prepared: how does one verify their concentrations? If one of these two products is available commercially as assayed material, the problem is reduced by analyzing one against the other. However, if neither can be purchased, I recommend the following steps:

1. Submit samples of controls and reference standards to a reference laboratory for analysis. Close communication with the reference laboratory is necessary; avoid submitting these samples as blind submissions. For example, instruct the reference laboratory to keep the sample frozen until ready for analysis, because this is the procedure used in day-to-day analysis. However, specifying the expected concentration of analyte is not necessary.

2. Plot a calibration curve after determining verified standards by the selected method of analysis.

3. Send 10 to 20 split samples from patients to a reference laboratory and compare the results. Again, communicate your intentions to the reference laboratory.

4. Finally, subscribers to proficiency test programs can purchase leftover samples, if available, which represent assayed material.

Internal Quality Assurance

After procuring the necessary materials and preparing quality-control samples and standards for analysis, a statistical protocol must be established to evaluate the results obtained. At this point in method development, the standards have been verified and analyzed numerous times in duplicate, and the quality-control samples have also been analyzed. As data begin to accumulate, the analyst is ready to apply the statistical methods chosen.

The methods chosen should be easy to handle daily as well as monthly. Sheets for data records should be convenient to the analysis site and stored in a notebook in some clearly identified location. A supervisor or laboratory director should review these records regularly.

The Shewhart (10) chart, introduced to clinical chemistry by Levey and Jennings (11) (Figure 1), is widely

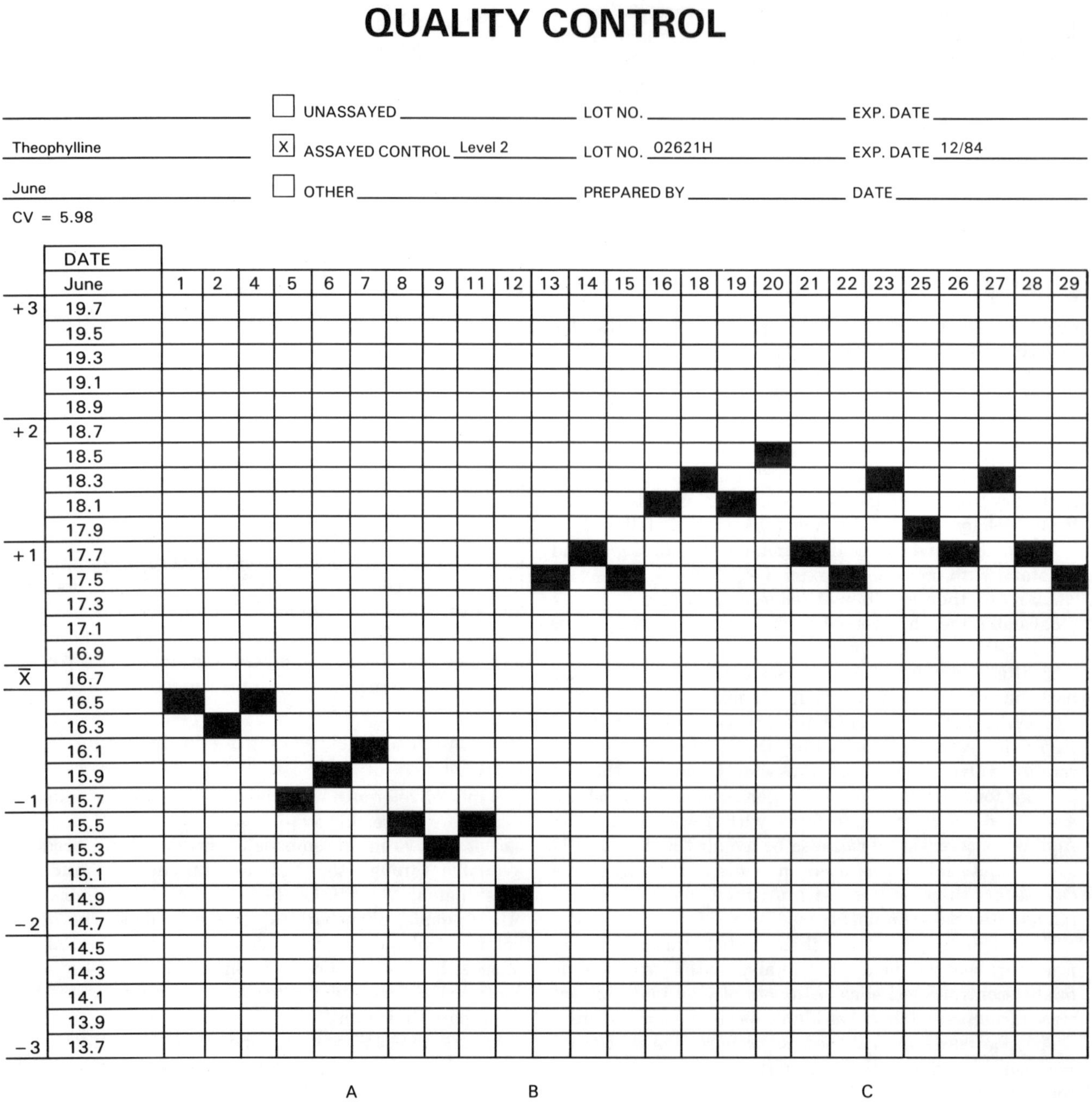

QUALITY CONTROL

Theophylline
June
CV = 5.98

[X] ASSAYED CONTROL Level 2 LOT NO. 02621H EXP. DATE 12/84

Fig. 1. Levey-Jennings control chart demonstrating: (A) a trend, (B) a shift, and (C) a change in the mean

used in clinical laboratories today (12). These charts are prepared by arranging the concentration on the ordinate to encompass values from $\bar{x} + 3s$ to $\bar{x} - 3s$. The abscissa is scaled to the time period of interest. For example, for daily analysis, one would scale this chart to be one month, but for analytes that are requested less often, greater intervals would be appropriate. Different horizontal lines correspond to $\bar{x} \pm 3s$, $\bar{x} \pm 2s$, and $\bar{x} \pm 1s$. Colors can be added to make the charts easier to review at month's end. For new quality-control material the value for s is not known; therefore, one can temporarily assume that the target value is the mean ($\bar{x}$) and calculate s by using an assigned CV. In the early stages of developing a method, one might assign CVs of 5%, 10%, and 15% as a starting point. In the final steps of development, the CV for a precise method (e.g., for lithium) should be less than 5%. Complex procedures that require multiple extractions might have a CV as great as 10%, especially if performed by several different technologists. When a CV exceeds 15%, the method should be deemed unacceptable, and either the method refined or another method sought, unless semiquantitative results are adequate for care of patients. Several commercial vendors of TDM control material provide laboratories with some form of personalized Levey-Jennings quality-control charts, with the limits already computed and labeled. These charts are then submitted monthly for interlaboratory comparisons.

Tonks (13) recommends calculating an "allowable limit of error" for clinical chemistry tests. This is a concept toxicologists could use in determining what CV will be tolerated. Obviously, one would expect the CV to be lower for an enzyme immunoassay for tobramycin than for a capillary gas-chromatographic assay for diazepam. When determining what CV is suitable, one should examine the therapeutic range of analytes and make decisions based on the potential for toxicity.

With the use of Levey-Jennings charts, a method can be monitored for trends, shifts, or changes in the mean (Figure 1). One can note on the charts the dates of reagent changes or instrument maintenance, the name of the technician performing the test, and the time of day of analysis. If one of these changes is responsible for a shift (Figure 1), the chart should reflect the problem. Trend analysis is especially important when a quality-control material is not available commercially and when the stability of the analyte in frozen serum has not been established. Through careful periodical preparation of reference standards, one can detect deterioration of quality-control material; however, if standards and quality-control materials are prepared at the same time and stored in the same freezer, they might deteriorate together at the same rate without being noticed.

Proficiency test samples are also useful monitors when no commercially assayed material is available.

Urine drug screening and other qualitative toxicology tests are more difficult to evaluate day-to-day and should therefore have more frequent quality-control assessment; for example, every TLC plate should include at least one quality-control sample along with standards and patients' samples. Give careful attention to changes in lot numbers of reagents or of extraction columns and in the volumes of sample used. When hundreds of urines are analyzed daily, subtle changes in procedures may easily occur and adversely affect results. Submission of blind test samples is the most effective way to monitor quality. Figure 2 shows one way that TLC results can be recorded.

Finally, what about an analysis the toxicologist is asked to perform only once? Consider the case when analysis of blood and urine samples from a comatose patient detected no drugs; however, a relative of the patient remembered that, just before becoming ill, the patient vomited on the sleeve of her coat. Careful extraction of the coat fabric indicated the presence of haloperidol but, because this was not one of the analytes the laboratory routinely tests for in blood or urine, there were no prepared standards or quality-control materials available. In this case the analysis should be done at least in duplicate, with another square of fabric from the coat (without vomit) serving as a blank. Mass spectroscopy, if available, is also desirable because of its specificity. Specimens like this, plus the blood and urine samples, should then be sent to a reference laboratory to confirm the presence of haloperidol.

Proficiency Testing Programs

Proficiency testing should be viewed as a fine-tuning mechanism, to be applied only after other components such as qualified personnel, adequate laboratory facilities, adherence to strict guidelines of method selection, and development of a functional internal quality-control program have been satisfactorily established.

Over the years, laboratories have responded favorably to interchanging specimens and comparing results with one another. These results enable a laboratory to evaluate its own performance critically and either increase its confidence in its methods or encourage a change to a better one. One of the drawbacks in many proficiency testing programs is the delay between submitting the test results and receiving the summary of survey results. Perhaps future analyses will overcome this problem by utilizing computers and telephone modems. Because licensure of laboratories is often influenced by quality-control results and performance with these samples, the laboratory supervisor is encouraged to submit proficiency test samples as unknowns instead of blind specimens. Unfortunately, unknowns do not truly reflect analytical performance obtained with patients' samples, which thus enables the laboratory to show a better performance. To add to this false sense of security, the night and evening shifts at the laboratory are seldom asked to analyze proficiency test specimens. Schwartz et al. (14) in 1978 reported that a pilot "blind" proficiency test program gave the following results: only 15 to 20% of the samples submitted to a night shift were successfully analyzed with acceptable results, compared with 70 to 75% correct results determined in the same laboratory during the day shift. Many reports in the literature reflect a change in performance when samples are submitted blind as patients' samples instead of as unknown samples.

Samples used for blind testing should be manufactured professionally or made by someone knowledgeable of manufacturing processes. The fact that an individual is an expert toxicologist does not qualify him or her to prepare samples for a quality-assurance program. For example, it is counterproductive and frustrating to assay specimens that contain unnatural amounts of drug and metabolites and that may be contaminated with bacteria.

Proficiency testing requirements were part of the Clinical Laboratory Improvement Act (CLIA) of 1967, a law that initiated the development of several new proficiency testing programs as part of licensing interstate laboratories. Established toxicology proficiency

THIN LAYER CHROMATOGRAPHY DATA SHEET

SPECIMEN INFORMATION

Sample I.D. Number _____

Date: _____

Specimen Type: _____

Analysis Done By: _____

COMMENTS:

QUALITY CONTROL: ANALYSIS DATA

ug/mL	DRUG	weak	mod	strong
1	Propoxyphene			
1	Normethadone			
1	Methadone			
1	Phencyclidine			
1	Methaqualone			
2	Meperidine			
4	Oxycodone			
2	Glutethimide			
3	Meprobamate			
2	Amphetamine			
2	Methamphetamine			
1	Phenobarbital			
1	Codeine			
1	Morphine			
4	Benzoylecgonine			

SAMPLE DATA

BASES

1) R_f _____ Spot Shape _____
   Visualization:
   stage 1:
   stage 2:
   stage 3:
   stage 4:
   Metabolites:

2) R_f _____ Spot Shape _____
   Visualization
   stage 1:
   stage 2:
   stage 3:
   stage 4:
   Metabolites:

SEDATIVES/HYPNOTICS

1) R_f _____ Spot Shape _____
   Visualization
   stage 1:
   stage 2:
   stage 3:
   stage 4:
   Metabolites

2) R_f _____ Spot Shape _____
   Visualization
   stage 1:
   stage 2:
   stage 3:
   stage 4:
   Metabolites:

USE ADDITIONAL SHEETS IF MORE COMPOUNDS ARE PRESENT

CONFIRMATORY DATA:

RESULTS TO BE REPORTED:

Fig. 2. Record sheet for emergency toxicology TLC drug screen in urine

Reprinted by permission of Accutox Laboratories, North Canton, OH

programs have now been available for more than a decade, the three most well-known having developed as follows:

The first program was started in 1972 by the Centers for Disease Control (CDC) (15), which had assumed the responsibility for implementing the CLIA. The toxicology programs available in 1972 included drugs of abuse, drug overdose, therapeutic drug monitoring, blood lead, and environmental poisons. Today only two toxicology programs are offered by the CDC Proficiency Testing Branch: blood lead and drug monitoring. Specimens are sent out quarterly and the service is free of charge.

In November 1972 the College of American Pathologists (CAP) initiated a survey called the Toxicology Evaluation Program. On the first submission, more than 40% of the participants failed to identify morphine in urine (16) at a concentration of 1.0 mg/L. Programs available now are TDM series 1 and 2, urine toxicology, and toxicology series 1 and 2. Specimens are sent quarterly to subscribers for a fee. The CAP continuing education program is not coordinated with the survey program.

The third source is the American Association for Clinical Chemistry (AACC), which offers programs in therapeutic drug monitoring and emergency toxicology. These comprehensive programs offer proficiency test specimens and continuing education material monthly. This program began in 1974 when Pippenger et al. (17,18) distributed samples containing anticonvulsant drugs to neurologists who were to submit them to their laboratories for analysis. The poor results obtained prompted the development of a proficiency survey program to assist laboratories in improving the quality of testing for anticonvulsant drugs.

Remember, quality-control charts reflect the performance a laboratory is capable of attaining in day-to-day practice. Professionally prepared proficiency test specimens submitted to the laboratory as unknown samples reflect the absolute best results the laboratory is capable of attaining. These same high-quality specimens submitted as blind specimens represent the actual performance of the laboratory. The majority of toxicologists willingly accept the challenge of a blind test program if it is executed properly and if the goal is to improve the quality of testing and not to provoke punitive measures.

Discussion

Only a decade ago, procedures for emergency toxicology analyses were run primarily in large hospitals and reference laboratories. The emergency room physician's wait for results forced treatment of symptoms only. Often, the results, received a few days later, came too late to affect treatment and simply became part of the patient's records. These analytical procedures are more widely available now with the introduction of enzyme immunoassays for many more drugs, simpler and better-defined TLC procedures, and the refinement of sophisticated instrumentation such as gas chromatography/mass spectroscopy.

The laboratory director who decides to offer a new toxicology service must confront the issue of standards and controls, an integral part of the quality-assurance program. The establishment of qualitative procedures (e.g., TLC screening for drugs of abuse) does not present any unusually difficult problems for quality control. Quantitative analysis, however, will require the preparation of quality-control samples because not all groups of drugs are available commercially. When a toxicology program is first started, quantitative results may not be offered because of inadequate instrumentation and staff training. However, a good toxicology service should eventually offer quantitative results. For example, to tell a physician in a trauma unit that barbiturates have been detected in a patient may be misleading if the amounts found were low and unrelated to the patient's condition. Often, even semiquantitative results are adequate.

Because of the large number of analytes capable of being stained and viewed in TLC procedures, the toxicologist may be tempted to increase the number of drugs to be detected. For an acceptable program, each analyte that the laboratory is responsible for detecting must be detected in at least one confirmation test to further prove its presence. Analytes listed as detectable in an new toxicology service should be limited to the drugs that are confirmed by techniques all the technologists are capable of performing. Additional analytes can be added as the acquisition of equipment and training of the staff allow.

Limits of detection for analytes are also very important. The desire for analysts to detect smaller amounts of drugs in smaller volumes of biological fluid has not gone without its rewards, including improved detection and economy of resources. However, when limits of detection are set, these should be realistic numbers and not established from other influences. When a laboratory indicates that it can detect morphine in urine at 0.5 mg/L, this should indicate a confirmed quantitative result and not simply the visualization of a spot with iodoplatinate reagent on a TLC plate. To monitor technique, extraction efficiencies, and TLC staining reagents, one should include a quality-control sample with analyte concentrations close to the detection limit with every group of samples assayed. These sample concentrations in urine, at or below detection limits, are also good training aids for new technologists learning toxicology procedures.

Proficiency testing, both external and internal, is one of the most important parts of a toxicology quality-assurance program. It can be a humbling experience to blind-test your own laboratory: one gets a deeper meaning of the phrase, "To err is human." Mason (19) reported poor performance on many CAP surveys; in fact, CVs greater than 30% were common, even though most of these samples were submitted to the laboratory as unknowns and not as blind samples. According to reports in the literature (14), less-than-desirable performance is the rule, not the exception, in surveys where samples are truly submitted blind, especially if all work shifts are included in the evaluation. Nonetheless, blind proficiency testing is necessary in the search for excellence. The key to an effective blind proficiency survey is the constructive use of the data gathered rather than punitive responses. Clinical chemistry has reached such a level of automation that performance in blind surveys reflects performance in determinations of unknowns. This is not true for toxicology, however, in which many procedures are left to human interpretation and decision.

The laboratory director should consider certain pitfalls when considering participation in a blind proficiency test. First is the problem of making the specimen appear authentic. Split specimens are a good source of "real" samples, but one must remember that these provide only a check on reproducibility, not accuracy, because both results could be wrong. Analytes with available metabolites (e.g., amitriptyline/nortriptyline) can be added to the matrix. However, unless the value of the added analyte had been verified by a reputable laboratory, these samples also are useful only in checking reproducibility. One of the best sources of specimen is leftover survey samples, or leftover samples from the stock of the vendor for the survey. If leftover samples are to be used, one should immediately after use divide them into aliquots in suitably marked containers and store them in a freezer. Treat all subsequent samples the same as the first, to rule out any changes in analyte that may occur because of the action of bacteria or the effect of standing at room temperature. If these samples are made from working standards of analyte, remove the alcohol to a clinically realistic concentration. For example, submitting a blind specimen containing 10 mL of methanol per liter is counterproductive in terms of the extra analytical time involved (and wasted), because this content represents severe toxicity. Analysts are not pleased about spending time on an improperly prepared specimen. The results of a blind survey should be available within a few days, especially when deficiencies are noted, so that corrective measures can be taken. Finally, quality reference laboratories conduct or participate in blind surveys and are usually willing to be of service for their clients.

With increasing demands on the laboratory and a need for faster turnaround time to shorten hospital stays, it is easy to ignore "avoidable" activities such as a toxicology quality-assurance program. However, in our efforts to assure the highest-quality results for patient care, we must maintain careful monitoring of daily analytical activity through assessing quality control.

References

1. Westgard JO, de Vos DJ, Hunt MR, et al. Concepts and practices in the evaluation of clinical chemistry methods, III: Statistics. *Am J Med Technol* **44**, 552-569 (1978).
2. Buttner J, Borth R, Boutwell JH, et al. Provisional recommendations on quality control in clinical chemistry. *Clin Chem* **22**, 532-540 (1976).
3. Evans JG. Legal aspects and regulations pertaining to sale and distribution of analytical standards for drugs of abuse. Part I. *J Chromatogr Sci* **10**, 342-346 (1972).
4. Johnson EL, Stevenson R. *Basic Liquid Chromatography*, Varian Associates Inc., Palo Alto, CA, 1978, 238 pp.
5. Thoma JJ. Quality assurance in toxicology. In *Guidelines for Analytical Toxicology Programs*, 1, JJ Thoma et al., Eds. CRC Press, Cleveland, OH, 1977, pp 133-167.
6. Finkle BS. Quality assurance in toxicology. *J Anal Toxicol* **7**, 158-160 (1983).
7. Proksch GJ, Bonderman DP. Preparation of optically clear lyophilized human serum for use in preparing control material. *Clin Chem* **22**, 456-460 (1976).
8. Fields PH, Basteyns BJ, Everson AM, et al. Clinical toxicology. In *Quality Assurance Practices for Health Care Laboratories*, SL Inhorn, Ed., Public Health Assoc., Washington, DC, 1978, pp 1033-1096.
9. Frings CS, Waldrop NT. Quality control in the toxicology laboratory. *Lab Med* **6**, 16-27 (1975).
10. Shewart WA. *Economic Control of Quality of the Manufactured Product*, Van Nostrand, New York, NY, 1931.
11. Levey S, Jennings ER. The use of control charts in the clinical laboratory. *Am J Clin Pathol* **20**, 1059-1066 (1950).
12. Westgard JO, Barry PL, Hunt MR, et al. A multi-rule Shewart chart for quality control in clinical chemistry. *Clin Chem* **27**, 493-501 (1981).
13. Tonks DB. A quality control program for quantitative clinical chemistry estimations. *Can J Med Technol* **30**, 38-54 (1968).
14. Schwartz MK, Blatt S, Blumenfeld TA. Clinical chemistry. *Op. cit.* (ref. 8), p 490.
15. Boone DJ, Guerrant GO, Knouse RW. Proficiency testing in clinical toxicology: Program sponsored by the Center for Disease Control. *J Anal Toxicol* **1**, 147-150 (1977).
16. Sohn D. The College of American Pathologists toxicology program. *Ibid.*, pp 111-117.
17. Pippenger CE, Paris-Kutt H, Penry JK, et al. Proficiency testing in determinations of antiepileptic drugs. *Ibid.*, pp 118-122.
18. Dijkhuis IC, DeJong HJ, Richens A, et al. Joint international quality control programme on the determination of antiepileptic drugs. *Pharm Weekblad* **114**, 1171-1204 (1979).
19. Mason MF. Some realities and results of proficiency testing of laboratories performing toxicological analysis. *J Anal Toxicol* **5**, 201-208 (1981).

Screening Procedures. I. Multiple Drugs by Thin-Layer Chromatography

Submitter: Larry A. Broussard, *Medical Laboratory Associates, Birmingham, AL 35256*

Evaluators: Ted W. Fendley and Linda Pellegrino, *International Clinical Labs, Lexington, KY 40503*

Introduction

The increasing use of pharmaceuticals in our daily lives has made necessary the confirmation of drug ingestion by the laboratory. Besides drug identification in possible overdoses, other needs include forensic reasons, employee screening, and monitoring surreptitious use of drugs. The specimen of choice for screening for most drugs is urine: the concentrations of many drugs are higher in urine than in blood, and there is generally enough sample for a complete examination.

Among the many methods for identifying drugs in urine—infrared spectroscopy, gas chromatography, radioimmunoassay, mass spectroscopy, immunoassays, ultraviolet spectroscopy—thin-layer chromatography (TLC) offers several advantages (*1-4*): a relatively small investment in equipment, the ability to analyze several samples simultaneously, simplicity, and sensitivity. TLC procedures involve extraction of drugs with resins or organic solvents, concentration by solvent evaporation, separation on a chromatographic plate, and identification by use of solutions or sprays. The method presented here, developed and modified by Frings and colleagues (*4*), has been used in our laboratory for 15 years to detect the following drugs in urine, gastric contents, pills, or capsules: amphetamines, phenylpropanolamine, chlorpheniramine, pseudoephedrine, phenmetrazine, methadone, meperidine, propoxyphene, codeine, hydromorphone, cocaine, morphine, glutethimide, barbiturates, meprobamate, tricyclic antidepressants (amitriptyline, nortriptyline, imipramine, desipramine, and doxepin), and phencyclidine. The procedure is easily adapted to identification of many other drugs of interest.

Principle

The drugs are extracted into chloroform/isobutanol (98/2 by vol) at pH 9.0 (±0.3), concentrated, and subjected to separation on three TLC plates.

Barbiturates, glutethimide, and meprobamate are detected as colored spots on one TLC plate after staining with mercurous nitrate, mercuric sulfate, diphenylcarbazone, and vanillin.

Most other drugs are detected on a second TLC plate. Amphetamines, phenylpropanolamine, pseudoephedrine, phenmetrazine, and the major metabolite(s) of methadone, meperidine, and chlorpheniramine are detected by staining with ninhydrin. Morphine, codeine, hydromorphone, phencyclidine, cocaine and its metabolite, and propoxyphene and its metabolite are detected by staining with an iodoplatinic acid reagent.

Codeine and tricyclic antidepressants are detected on a third TLC plate.

Materials and Methods

Reagents

1. *Borate buffer, pH 9.3*: Mix 950 mL of a filtered, saturated sodium borate solution with 50 mL of 0.3 mol/L NaOH (12.0 g of NaOH per liter). Measure the pH and adjust to pH 9.3 (±0.05) with saturated sodium borate solution or 0.3 mol/L NaOH. Stable for three months when stored at room temperature.

2. *Chloroform/isobutanol mixture (98/2, by vol)*: Stable for two weeks when stored in a brown glass bottle at room temperature.

3. *0.1 mol/L HCl in methanol*: Add 0.8 mL of concentrated HCl to methanol in a 100-mL volumetric flask and dilute to volume with methanol. Stable for three months when stored in a brown bottle at room temperature.

4. *Barbiturate developing solvent*: Just before use, mix 99 mL of chloroform and 11 mL of acetone. Use this reagent only once and discard.

5. *Alkaloid developing solvent*: Just before use, mix 84 mL of ethyl acetate, 35 mL of absolute ethanol, 5 mL of *n*-butanol, and 0.6 mL of concentrated NH_4OH (cat. no. 3256-1; Mallinckrodt, Inc., Paris, KY 40301). Use this reagent only once and discard.

6. *Barbiturate and glutethimide detection reagent*: Just before use, prepare a saturated solution of mercurous nitrate by shaking 0.5 g of $HgNO_3 \cdot H_2O$ in 50 mL of water for 2 to 3 min. Vials or tubes containing 0.5 g of $HgNO_3 \cdot H_2O$ may be prepared ahead of time and stored for daily use.

7. *$HgSO_4$ reagent*: Suspend, with mixing, 5.0 g of HgO (mercuric oxide) in 100 mL of water in a 250-mL volumetric flask. Add, with mixing, 20 mL of concentrated H_2SO_4. Cool and dilute to 250 mL with water. Stable for one month when stored in a brown bottle at room temperature.

8. *Diphenylcarbazone reagent*: Dissolve 5 mg of diphenylcarbazone in 50 mL of $CHCl_3$. Stable for one month when stored in a brown glass bottle at room temperature.

9. *Ninhydrin reagent*: Dissolve 0.2 g of ninhydrin in 50 mL of *n*-butanol. Use within 2 h after preparation. Vials or

tubes containing 0.2 g of ninhydrin may be prepared and stored for daily use.

10. *HCl, 2 mol/L*: Add 167 mL of concentrated HCl to approximately 600 mL of water in a 1-L volumetric flask and dilute to volume with water. Stable for one year when stored at room temperature.

11. *Stock iodoplatinic acid reagent*: Transfer 4.5 g of KI and 10 mL of chloroplatinic acid ($H_2PtCl_6 \cdot 6H_2O$) solution (50 g/L) to a 200-mL Erlenmeyer flask. Add 100 mL of water and dissolve the KI. Stable for one month when stored at 2-6 °C in a brown glass bottle.

12. *Working iodoplatinic acid reagent*: Mix stock reagent with an equal volume of 2 mol/L HCl. Use within 3 h after preparation.

13. *Vanillin reagent*: Dissolve 0.5 g of vanillin in methanol and dilute to 50 mL with methanol. Add 1.0 mL of concentrated H_2SO_4 and mix. Prepare fresh reagent each day. Vials or tubes containing 0.5 g of vanillin may be prepared and stored for daily use.

14. *Mecke's reagent*: Dissolve 0.50 g of selenious acid (no. A-286; Fisher Scientific Co., Fair Lawn, NJ) in 100 mL of concentrated H_2SO_4. Stable for one month when stored in a brown bottle at room temperature.

15. *T1, tricyclic antidepressant standard (doxepin, 4 mg/L)*: Dissolve 18.1 mg of doxepin hydrochloride (Pfizer Laboratories, New York, NY 10017) in about 50 mL of methanol and dilute to exactly 4000 mL with water. Stable for one year when stored frozen, or three months when stored at 2-6 °C.

16. *T2, tricyclic antidepressant standard (amitriptyline, nortriptyline, imipramine, and desipramine, 4 mg/L each)*: Dissolve 18.1 mg of amitriptyline hydrochloride (Merck, Sharpe & Dohme, West Point, PA 19486), 18.2 mg of nortriptyline hydrochloride (Eli Lilly & Co., Indianapolis, IN 46285), 18.1 mg of imipramine hydrochloride (Geigy Pharmaceuticals, Ardsley, NY 10502), and 18.1 mg of desipramine hydrochloride (Merrell-National Laboratories, Cincinnati, OH 45215) in about 100 mL of methanol and dilute to exactly 4000 mL with water. Stable for one year when stored frozen or three months when stored at 2-6 °C.

17. *Phencyclidine standard, 5 mg/L*: Dissolve 5.4 mg of phencyclidine hydrochloride (Philips Roxane, Inc., St. Joseph, MO 64502) in water and dilute to volume in a 1-L volumetric flask. Stable for six months when stored in a brown glass bottle at 2-6 °C.

18. *Urine drug control, levels 1 and 2*: a. Collect 8 L of drug-free urine for each control to be prepared. It is desirable to freeze the urine until enough urine is obtained to proceed with the rest of the procedure.

b. Filter the urine through glass wool.

c. Weigh the following amounts (milligrams) of each drug and place each drug in a separate test tube (see *Notes*).

	Control 1	Control 2
Morphine · HCl[a]	20.8	31.2
Codeine · SO_4[a]	41.6	31.2
Methadone · HCl[b]	17.7	26.6
Methamphetamine · HCl[c]	19.8	29.7
Phenobarbital, sodium[a]	17.6	26.4
Secobarbital, sodium[d]	17.4	26.1
Amphetamine · HCl[c]	30.3	45.5
Phenmetrazine · HCl[e]	38.4	57.6
Propoxyphene · HCl[d]	17.7	26.2
Meprobamate[f]	64.0	96.0

[a] Merck & Co., Inc., Rahway, NJ.
[b] Mallinckrodt Chemical Works, St. Louis, MO.
[c] Sigma Chemical Co., St. Louis, MO.
[d] Eli Lilly & Co., St. Louis, MO.
[e] Ciba Pharmaceutical Co., Summit, NJ.
[f] Wyeth Laboratories, Philadelphia, PA.

d. Add approximately 2 mL of water to each tube and dissolve the drugs.

e. Dissolve 70.4 mg (Control 1) and 105.6 mg (Control 2) of cocaine · HCl (Merck) in separate 100-mL solutions of saturated Na_3BO_3 and let stand five days at room temperature.

f. Suspend a 125-mg tablet of glutethimide (Doriden; USV Pharmaceutical Corp., Tuckahoe, NY 10707) in 125 mL of absolute ethanol, mix well, and filter. Use 16.0 mL (Control 1) and 24 mL (Control 2) of this filtered solution.

g. Pipet 0.90 mL (44.9 mg, Control 1) and 1.4 mL (70 mg, Control 2) of meperidine · HCl (50 mg/mL; Winthrop Labs., New York, NY) into two tubes.

h. Pipet 8.8 mL (17.9 mg, Control 1) and 13.4 mL (26.8 mg, Control 2) of hydromorphone · HCl (Dilaudid · HCl, 2 mg/mL; Knoll Pharmaceutical Co., Whippany, NJ) into two tubes.

i. Place about 1500 mL of filtered urine (from step *b*) in a 2-L volumetric flask.

j. Add the Control 1 set of dissolved drugs to this urine. Rinse each tube with urine to assure complete transfer of the drugs.

k. Dilute the contents of the 2-L volumetric flask to volume with urine and mix well.

l. Transfer this urine to a container that will hold and allow mixing of 8 L of urine.

m. Measure and transfer 2-L aliquots of drug-free urine to this container until the total 8 L has been transferred.

n. Mix the urine with a magnetic stirrer for about 2 h.

o. Measure the pH of the urine drug control. If it is greater than 7.0, adjust the pH to 6.0-7.0 with concentrated HCl.

p. Transfer the urine drug control to suitable containers. Assign a lot number and date. Stable for six months at 2-6 °C, or 15 months when stored frozen.

q. Repeat steps *i-p* for the set of drugs for Control 2.

Notes: 1. For a laboratory to obtain many of the drugs listed, a Controlled Substances Registration Certificate must be obtained. Inquiries concerning the application procedure for this certificate for an analytical laboratory should be addressed to: United States Department of Justice, Drug Enforcement Administration, Washington, DC 20537. Applicants should anticipate that this process may be lengthy, owing to the nature of the agency involved and the implications of such a certificate.

2. The amount of each drug used is calculated on the basis of the free base form of each drug. The final concentration (mg/L) of each drug in the urine controls is as follows:

	Control 1	Control 2
Amphetamine	3	4.5
Cocaine (converted to benzoylecgonine)	8	12
Glutethimide	2	3
Hydromorphone	2	3
Meperidine	4	6
Meprobamate	4	6
Methadone	2	3
Methamphetamine	2	3
Morphine	2	3
Phenmetrazine	4	6
Phenobarbital	2	3
Propoxyphene	2	3
Secobarbital	2	3

3. If an amount of control other than 8 L is to be prepared, then the amounts of each drug listed in steps c-n must be changed to agree with the final concentrations listed above.

4. Evaluators T.W.F. and L.P. report that they save considerable time by dissolving all of the drugs used in their control materials in approximately 10 mL of reagent-grade ethanol and mixing in urine for several hours.

Apparatus

1. *Extraction tubes:* The following 50-mL polypropylene tubes have been checked and found to be acceptable for use in this procedure: 50-mL polypropylene lab tube (Medical Polymers, Inc., Canton, MA 02021). Acceptable for the extraction procedure only (steps 1-6 in the procedure) are 50-mL polypropylene centrifuge tubes with polyethylene caps (cat. no. 8889-205137; Lancer, St. Louis, MO 63103). Before using any tubes other than these, check to verify their acceptability.

   Note: On occasion, some lots of these (particularly the first kind) or other tubes give artifactual spots on the TLC plates (usually a gray spot interfering with the glutethimide spots, or a white spot interfering with the barbiturates on the barbiturate plate, or a yellowish spot near the solvent front on the alkaloid plate). When these artifacts have been observed, the tubes have looked opaque instead of clear. The artifacts are apparently unknown compounds leached from the tubes during solvent evaporation (procedure step 9).

2. *TLC plates:* The Submitter uses LK5DF plates (cat. no. 4856-821; Whatman Chemical Separation, Inc., Clifton, NJ 07014) divided into 19 channels. The lower, pre-absorbent region on these plates allows the analyst to rapidly spot (streak) each sample onto a separate channel.

   Note: Each lot no. of plates should be checked before routine use to ensure that the characteristic migration patterns of the drugs described in the interpretation sections are seen. Rarely, some lots of plates will incompletely or inadequately separate the drugs. Such plates should be exchanged for another lot number. If this is impossible, slight modification of the composition of the developing solvent may yield satisfactory migration patterns.

3. *Chromatography tanks:* The Submitter uses rectangular (30 × 9.8 × 25 cm, $l \times w \times h$) molded glass tanks (cat. no. 05-718-16; Fisher Scientific, Pittsburgh, PA 15219) with flat glass lids.

4. *Sprayer:* Attach an air sprayer (e.g., Bink's Model 59-10001A, available at hobby or craft shops) to the laboratory compressed-air system via a regulator and shut-off valve. Routinely, the air pressure used is about 345 kPa (50 lb./in.^{2}). Aspirate the reagents to be sprayed from 75 × 100 mm disposable glass test tubes. Because of the corrosive nature of the sprays, aspirate water through the sprayer between each spray. Disassemble the sprayer and clean it sonically at least once weekly.

Other apparatus available for spraying reagents are available, including aerosol-powered sprayers (e.g., Chromist®, cat. no. 51901; Gelman Instrument Co., Ann Arbor, MI) or aspiration-type glass sprayers (cat. no. 5-8005; Supelco, Inc., Bellefonte, PA 16823-0048). The particular apparatus must be capable of evenly dispensing reagents of various viscosities (including the highly viscous Mecke's reagent) in a fine mist or in a saturating spray. The apparatus should also be durable and resistant to corrosive materials.

Procedure for Urine Samples

1. Add 15 mL of T1 and T2, urine drug control 1, urine drug control 2, tricyclic standards, and phencyclidine standard, to separate 50-mL glass-stoppered centrifuge tubes or 50-mL polypropylene tubes. Label as Control 1, Control 2, T1, T2, and PCP.

2. Add 15 mL of urine sample to another 50-mL tube, labeled unknown.

3. Add 3.0 mL of pH 9.3 borate buffer to each tube.

4. Add 25 mL of chloroform/isobutanol (98/2, by vol) mixture to each tube.

   Note: Automated pipets or dispensers are convenient for steps 3, 4, and 8.

5. Shake tubes for 5 min on a mechanical shaker or invert at least 20 times.

6. Aspirate the aqueous (upper) layer and discard. If an emulsion forms, add 0.5 to 1.0 mL of methanol and mix well again; if necessary, the tubes may be centrifuged to separate the layers.

7. Filter the chloroform (bottom) layer through Whatman no. 1 filter paper into appropriately labeled 50-mL tubes.

8. Add 0.1 mL of HCl, 0.1 mol/L in methanol, to each tube.

9. Evaporate extracts at 50-65 °C under a stream of dry air in a fume hood.

10. Dissolve the residue from each extract in 100 µL of methanol, with vortex-mixing, and stopper the tubes tightly.

Procedure for Gastric Contents

Gastric specimens are extracted by the same procedures as urine specimens except that pre-extraction with hexane is included. Urine drug control 1 is used as the control and is also taken through the hexane pre-extraction procedure.

1. Add 15 mL of gastric contents and urine drug control 1 to separate 50-mL polypropylene tubes or to glass centrifuge tubes.

2. Add two drops of concentrated HCl to each sample.

3. Using pH paper, check the pH. If the pH is >2, add concentrated HCl dropwise until the pH is <2.

4. Add 15 mL of hexane and shake vigorously.

5. Allow to settle. Centrifuge, if necessary, to separate layers.

6. Aspirate the hexane (top) layer and discard.

7. Add 3.0 mL of borate buffer and mix.

8. Check the pH. If it is about 9.0 (±0.5), proceed with the drug screen extraction procedure detailed above for urine. If the pH is too acidic, add 5 mol/L NaOH dropwise until the pH is 9.3, then proceed with the drug extraction procedure.

Procedure for Samples of Pills and Capsules

1. If only one pill or capsule is available, divide it into two pieces. If more than one pill is available, use separate pills in the following steps.

2. Dissolve one or one-half pill or capsule in about 1 mL (or less, depending on the solubility of the sample) of methanol. Spot this solution directly onto one set of three TLC plates, as described in step 1 of the TLC procedure (below).

3. Dissolve one or one-half pill or capsule in about 15 mL of water. Extract 15 mL of this solution as the unknown in step 2 of the extraction procedure for urine specimens.

TLC Procedure

1. Using a 50- or 100-µL Hamilton syringe, apply (streak) 20 µL of each reconstituted residue of control 1, control 2, T1, T2, and unknown to one TLC plate (the

Table 1. Summary of the Reaction of Drugs Tested with the Detection Reagents (X = positive reaction)

	Mercurous nitrate	Mercuric sulfate	Diphenyl-carbazone	Vanillin	Ninhydrin	Iodoplatinate
Acetaminophen (Tylenol)						
Acetophenetidine (Phenacetin)						
Amitriptyline HCl (Elavil)					X	X
Amobarbital, sodium	X	X	X			
Amphetamine HCl					X	
Amphetamine sulfate					X	
Benzoylecgonine (cocaine metabolite)						X
Benztropine mesylate (Cogentin)						X
Bromide, sodium						
Butabarbital, sodium	X	X	X			
Carisoprodol (Soma)						
Chloral hydrate						
Chlordiazepoxide (Librium)						X
Chloroquine (Aralen)						X
Chlorpheniramine maleate (Chlor-Trimeton)						X
Chlorpromazine HCl (Thorazine)		X		X		X
Clorazepate dipotassium (Tranxene)				X		X
Cocaine HCl						X
Codeine sulfate				X		X
Diazepam (Valium)						X
Diethylpropion HCl (Tenuate)						X
Diphenhydramine HCl (Benadryl)						X
Doxepin HCl (Sinequan)						X
Ephedrine HCl						
Ethchlorvynol (Placidyl)						
Ethinamate (Valmid)	X	X	X			
Fluphenazine HCl (Prolixin)		X		X		X
Flurazepam HCl (Dalmane)						X
Glutethimide (Doriden)	X		X			
Glycopyrrolate (Robinul)						
Haloperidol (Haldol)						X
Hydromorphone HCl (Dilaudid)						X
Imipramine HCl (Tofranil)		X		X		X
Mebutamate (Capla)						
Meperidine HCl (Demerol)						X
Mephenesin (Tolserol)				X		
Mephenesin carbamate (Tolseram)				X		
Meprobamate				X		
Methadone HCl						X
Methamphetamine HCl					X	
Methapyrilene HCl (Sominex)				X		X
Methaqualone (Sopor)						X
Methdilazine HCl (Tacaryl)		X		X		X
Methylphenidate HCl (Ritalin)						X
Methyprylon (Noludar)						
Morphine HCl						X

Table 1. (cont.)

	Mercurous nitrate	Mercuric sulfate	Diphenyl-carbazone	Vanillin	Ninhydrin	Iodoplatinate
Oxazepam (Serax)						
Oxycodone (Percodan)						X
Oxymetazoline (Afrin)						X
Pentazocine HCl (Talwin)						X
Pentobarbital	X	X	X			
Perphenazine (Trilafon)		X		X		X
Phencyclidine HCl (PCP)						X
Phenmetrazine HCl (Preludin)					X	X
Phenobarbital	X	X	X			
Phenylephrine HCl						
Phenylpropanolamine HCl					X	X
Phenytoin (Dilantin)	X	X	X			
Primaquine phosphate	X			X	X	X
Procainamide HCl (Pronestyl)						
Prochlorperazine edisylate (Compazine)		X		X		X
Promazine HCl (Sparine)		X		X		X
Promethazine HCl (Phenergan)		X		X		X
Propoxyphene HCl (Darvon)						X
Pseudoephedrine					X	X
Pyrilamine maleate						X
Pyrimethamine (Daraprim)	X					X
Quinidine sulfate						X
Quinine HCl						X
Salicylate sodium						
Scopolamine HCl						X
Secobarbital	X	X	X			
Strychnine sulfate						X
Sulfanilamide	X			X		
Tetracycline						
Thiobarbituric acid						
Thiopropazate HCl (Dartal)		X		X		X
Thioridazine HCl (Mellaril)		X		X		X
Thiothixene 2 HCl (Navane)				X		X
Trifluoperazine 2 HCl (Stelazine)		X		X		X
Triflupromazine HCl (Vesprin)		X		X		X
Trihexyphenidyl HCl (Artane)						X
Trimethobenzamide HCl (Tigan)						X
Trimethoxyphenethylamine HCl (mescaline)					X	
Tybamate (Solacen)						

barbiturate plate) and 30 μL to another plate (the alkaloid plate). Apply (streak) the remaining reconstituted residue to a third plate, labeled codeine. For PCP determinations, spot all of the reconstituted residue of the unknown and the PCP standard on the alkaloid plate. Whenever possible, the two outside channels on each plate should be left vacant. When running more than one set of three TLC drug plates, the order of specimens on the first set of alkaloid and codeine plates should be urine control 1, T1, T2, seven unknowns, urine drug control 2, and six unknowns; on all succeeding plates, T1 and T2 can be replaced with unknowns.

2. Place the barbiturate TLC plate in a chromatography tank that has been allowed to equilibrate for at least 15 min with barbiturate developing solvent (reagent no. 4).

3. Place the alkaloid TLC plate and the codeine TLC plate in a chromatography tank that has been allowed to equilibrate for at least 15 min with alkaloid developing solvent (reagent no. 5).

4. Allow the solvent in each chromatography tank to migrate about 8 cm up the TLC plate.

5. Remove the TLC plates from the tanks, immediately mark the solvent front with a pencil, then dry the plates in a 100 °C (± 10 °C) oven for 5 to 10 min.

Drug Detection: Barbiturate Plate

1. Pour the freshly prepared barbiturate and glutethimide detecting reagent (saturated $HgNO_3$) into a large dish and gently immerse the TLC plate in the solution, adsorbent side up.

2. Remove the plate, place it adsorbent side up on a paper towel, and look for gray spots.

Interpretation: The Rf of gray spots from the unknown should be compared with the Rf of barbiturates and glutethimide in Control 1 and Control 2. Spots in the unknown with the same Rf as glutethimide in the controls should be outlined in pencil for confirmation in the subsequent detection steps. Table 1 summarizes the reaction of all drugs tested with all the detection reagents used in this Selected Method. Table 2 lists the drugs that react with the mercurous nitrate reagent to form gray spots.

3. Dry the TLC plate in a 100 °C oven for 5 to 10 min.

4. Spray the TLC plate *very heavily* with $HgSO_4$ reagent. *Use a fume hood.*

Interpretation: The Rf of white spots from the unknown should be compared with the Rf of barbiturates in the controls. Table 3 lists drugs that react with the mercuric sulfate reagent. Those white spots in the unknown that correspond to or are between the Rfs of phenobarbital and secobarbital in the controls should be outlined in pencil to be confirmed with the diphenylcarbazone reagent.

5. Dry the TLC plate somewhat with a hair dryer or allow to airdry.

6. Spray *heavily* with diphenylcarbazone reagent. *Use a fume hood.*

Interpretation: Barbiturates and glutethimide reappear as blue or purple spots. Table 4 lists those drugs that react with the diphenylcarbazone reagent.

7. Place the TLC plate in a 100 °C oven for 3 to 5 min.

8. Remove, then spray the plate lightly with vanillin reagent.

9. Place the plate back in a 100 °C oven for 3 to 5 min.

10. Remove the plate from the oven and look for yellow spots.

Interpretation: A yellow spot corresponding to the same Rf as the yellow spot in Control 1 and Control 2 is positive for meprobamate. Table 5 lists those drugs that react with vanillin reagent.

Table 2. Migration Ratios[a] for Drugs Reacting with Mercurous Nitrate Reagent on Barbiturate TLC Plate

	R_G
Amobarbital, sodium	0.66
Butabarbital, sodium	0.54
Ethinamate	0.86
Glutethimide	1.00
Pentobarbital, sodium	0.65
Phenobarbital, sodium	0.46
Phenytoin	0.46
Primaquine phosphate	0.0
Pyrimethamine	0.0
Secobarbital, sodium	0.65
Sulfanilamide	0.20

[a] $R_G = \dfrac{\text{Distance drug migrates from point of application}}{\text{Distance glutethimide migrates from point of application}}$

Table 3. Characteristics of Drugs Reacting with Mercuric Sulfate Reagent on Barbiturate TLC Plate

	R_P[a]	Color
Amobarbital, sodium	1.5	White
Butabarbital, sodium	1.2	White
Chlorpromazine HCl	0.3	Pink
Ethinamate	2.0	White
Fluphenazin HCl	0.3	Orange
Imipramine HCl	0.3	Blue
Methdilazine HCl	0.3	Pink-orange
Pentobarbital, sodium	1.4	White
Perphenazine	0.3	Pink
Phenobarbital, sodium	1.0	White
Phenytoin	1.0	White
Prochlorperazine	0.3	Orange
Promazine HCl	0.3	Orange
Promethazine HCl	0.3	Pink-orange
Secobarbital, sodium	1.4	White
Thiopropazate HCl	0.3	Pink-orange
Thioridazine HCl	0.3	Blue
Trifluoperazine 2 HCl	0.3	Orange
Triflupromazine HCl	0.3	Orange

[a] $R_P = \dfrac{\text{Distance drug migrates from point of application}}{\text{Distance phenobarbital migrates from point of application}}$

Table 4. Characteristics of Drugs Reacting with Diphenylcarbazone Reagent on Barbiturate TLC Plate

	R_P[a]	Color
Amobarbital, sodium	1.5	Purple
Butabarbital, sodium	1.2	Purple
Ethinamate	2.0	Blue
Glutethimide	2.2	Purple
Pentobarbital, sodium	1.4	Purple
Phenobarbital, sodium	1.0	Purple
Phenytoin	1.0	Purple
Secobarbital, sodium	1.4	Purple

[a] See Table 3.

Drug Detection: Alkaloid Plate

1. Spray the TLC plate with freshly prepared ninhydrin reagent. *Use a fume hood.*

2. Dry the TLC plate in a 100 °C oven for 5 min.

3. Place the TLC plate under a short-wavelength ultraviolet lamp for 5 min, then record the visible spots.

Interpretation: Table 6 lists the drugs that react with ninhydrin. A pink spot corresponding to the same Rf as the red spots of amphetamine or methamphetamine in the controls should be confirmed for amphetamine. The major metabolite of methadone is detected as a pink spot. The major metabolite of meperidine is detected as a blue spot and is to be confirmed. Phenylpropanolamine is detected as a pink or red spot with an Rf between those for amphetamine and methamphetamine. Pseudoephedrine is detected as a red spot with an Rf slightly less than that of methamphetamine. Phenmetrazine is detected as a pink spot having the same Rf as the pink spot in Controls 1 and 2. The metabolites of chlorpheniramine are detected as two bluish-purple spots with Rfs less than that of methamphetamine.

When the sample to be analyzed is gastric contents, pills, or capsules, the interpretation of the plate for certain drugs is different because of the absence of metabolites.

4. Spray the TLC sheet with freshly prepared working iodoplatinic acid reagent. *Use a fume hood.*

Interpretation: Table 7 lists the drugs that react with the iodoplatinic acid reagent. The Rf of colored spots from the unknown should be compared with the Rf of morphine, hydromorphone, codeine, methadone, propoxyphene, and cocaine and its metabolite in Controls 1 and 2. Codeine and the tricyclic antidepressants may be identified by their colored spots at the Rf of these drugs in Controls 1 and 2 (codeine) and T1 and T2 (tricyclics) on both the alkaloid and codeine plates. Amphetamines from the unknown are identified by the fact that the spot(s) do not take up color when sprayed with the working iodoplatinic acid. The metabolites of diphenhydramine hydrochloride (Benadryl) may give a false-positive result for amphetamines. A reddish-purple spot at the same Rf as the reddish-purple spot on the PCP standard is positive for phenylcyclidine.

The metabolite of meperidine remains bluish-purple after spraying with the iodoplatinic reagent and should be reported as positive only if the unknown contains *both* the metabolite and a purple spot at the same Rf as the meperidine spot in Controls 1 and 2. Propoxyphene may be identified by the presence of its metabolite, which appears as a bluish smear; this characteristic color may fade (and reappear) when heated with a hair dryer. Phenylpropanolamine and pseudoephedrine have a characteristic reddish-orange color when sprayed with the iodoplatinic reagent. The metabolites of chlorpheniramine remain bluish-purple when sprayed with the reagent and the phenmetrazine spot remains pink.

When the sample to be analyzed is gastric contents, pills, or capsules, the interpretation of the plate for certain drugs is different because of the absence of metabolites.

Drug Detection: Codeine Plate

1. Place the plate in an oven (100 °C) for approximately 5 min.
2. Spray the codeine plate with Mecke's reagent.

Interpretation: A blue to green spot with the same Rf as the blue to green spot on the Controls 1 and 2 for codeine is codeine. If the blue to green spot does not appear, report as none detected for codeine. The presence of codeine may be confirmed by comparison with the codeine spot in Controls 1 and 2 on the alkaloid plate after it has been sprayed with the working iodoplatinic reagent. Observe the plate for spots in the unknowns corresponding to the same Rf as the spots in T1 and T2. The presence of the tricyclic antidepressants may be confirmed by comparison with the spots in T1 and T2 on the alkaloid plate after it has been sprayed with the working iodoplatinic reagent.

Results and Discussion

Interpretation and Specificity

The interpretation of the results for each plate used in this system is based on the comparison of the migration (Rf) and staining properties of the unknown spots on the plate with those of the standards or controls containing the drugs to be identified. Drug identification relies not only on the appreciation of the color characteristics and location of the spots on the plate but also on the experience of the analyst performing the interpretation. Tables 1 through 7 give pertinent information as to the specificity of the system for many drugs (4). In addition to the drugs listed here, the analyst should be aware that metabolites of drugs may also interfere with the interpretation process and that for many drugs (i.e., the benzodiazepines, methaqualone, and the phenothiazines) very little metabolized drug is present in the urine.

Analysts desiring to use this system to screen routinely for drugs other than those listed should do so only after

Table 5. Characteristics of Drugs Reacting with Vanillin Reagent on Barbiturate TLC Plate

	$R_M{}^a$	Color
Chlorpromazine HCl	0.6	Pink
Clorazepate dipotassium	3.8	Yellow
Codeine sulfate	1.5	Purple
Fluphenazin HCl	0.4	Orange
Imipramine HCl	0.8	Blue-green
Mephenesin carbamate	1.7	Pink-orange
Meprobamate	1.0	Yellow
Methapyrilene HCl	2.5	Purple
Methdilazine HCl	0.6	Pink
Perphenazine	0.6	Pink
Primaquine phosphate	2.5	Orange
Prochlorperazine edisylate	0.6	Pink
Promazine HCl	0.4	Orange
Promethazine HCl	0.4	Pink
Sulfanilamide	1.7	Yellow
Thiopropazate HCl	0.8	Pink
Thioridazine HCl	0.6	Violet
Thiothixene 2 HCl	0.8	Orange
Trifluoperazine 2 HCl	0.4	Orange
Triflupromazine HCl	0.4	Orange

$^a R_M = \dfrac{\text{Distance drug migrates from point of application}}{\text{Distance meprobamate migrates from point of application}}$

Table 6. Migration Ratios^a of Drugs Reacting with Ninhydrin Reagent on Alkaloid TLC Plate

	R_A
Amphetamine sulfate	1.00
Amitriptyline	1.47
Chlorpheniramine metabolites	0.40, 0.14
Desipramine	0.57
Diethylpropion HCl metabolite	1.4
Doxepin	1.33
Flurazepam HCl metabolite	1.0
Imipramine	1.28
Methadone metabolite	1.4
Methamphetamine HCl	0.80
Nortriptyline	0.78
Phencyclidine phosphate	2.09
Phenmetrazine HCl	1.1
Phenylpropanolamine	0.83
Primaquine phosphate	0.59
Pseudoephedrine	0.57
Trimethoxyphenethylamine HCl	0.59

$^a R_A = \dfrac{\text{Distance drug migrates from point of application}}{\text{Distance amphetamine migrates from point of application}}$

Table 7. Characteristics of Drugs Reacting with Iodoplatinic Reagent on Alkaloid TLC Plate

Drug	R_{Mo}[a]	Color	Drug	R_{Mo}[a]	Color
Amitriptyline HCl	2.4	Reddish-purple	Morphine HCl	1.0	Blue
Benzoylecgonine	0.1	Purple	Nicotine	2.4	Blue
Benztropine mesylate	0.8	Purple	Nortriptyline	1.3	Purple
Chlordiazepoxide	3.1	Reddish-purple	Oxycodone	2.5	Purple
Chloroquine phosphate	1.4	Purple	Oxymetazoline	0.5	Gray
Chlorpheniramine maleate	1.4	Purple	Pentazocine HCl	2.6	Reddish-purple
Chlorpheniramine metabolites	0.7	Bluish-purple	Perphenazine	2.0	Purple
Chlorpromazine HCl	2.5	Purple	Phenmetrazine HCl	1.8	Pink
Clorazepate dipotassium	3.5	Purple	Phenylpropanolamine	1.4	Reddish-orange
Cocaine HCl	3.5	Purple	Primaquine phosphate	1.1	Pink
Codeine sulfate	1.4	Purple	Prochlorperazine edisylate	1.9	Purple
Desipramine	0.9	Purple	Promazine HCl	2.1	Purple
Diazepam	3.5	Purple	Promethazine HCl	2.4	Purple
Diethylpropion HCl	3.1	Purple	Propoxyphene HCl	3.5	Purple
Diphenhydramine HCl	2.7	Reddish-purple	Pseudoephedrine	0.9	Reddish-orange
Doxepin HCl	2.2	Purple	Pyrilamine maleate	2.5	Purple
Fluphenazin HCl	2.2	Purple	Pyrimethamine	2.9	Purple
Flurazepam HCl	3.3	Purple	Quinidine sulfate	2.1	Purple
Flurazepam HCl metabolite	1.8	Purple	Quinine HCl	1.8	Purple
Haloperidol	3.4	Purple	Scopolamine HCl	2.3	Purple
Hydromorphone HCl	0.6	Purple	Strychnine sulfate	0.9	Purple
Imipramine HCl	2.1	Purple	Thiopropazate HCl	1.9, 3.2	Purple
Meperidine HCl	2.4	Reddish-purple	Thioridazine HCl	2.6	Purple
Methadone HCl	3.0	Reddish-purple	Thiothixene 2 HCl	1.7	Reddish-purple
Methapyrilene HCl	2.6	Purple	Trifluoperazine 2 HCl	2.0	Purple
Methaqualone	3.6	Purple	Triflupromazine HCl	2.9	Purple
Methdilazine HCl	1.5	Purple	Trihexyphenidyl HCl	3.7	Reddish-purple
Methylphenidate HCl	2.9	Purple	Trimethobenzamide HCl	2.1	Reddish-purple

[a] $R_{Mo} = \dfrac{\text{Distance drug migrates from point of application}}{\text{Distance morphine migrates from point of application}}$

investigating the suitability of the system for that use, e.g., by including the drugs of interest in appropriate standards or controls. Urine-based controls must be used whenever the migration pattern of a drug in urine differs from that of an aqueous standard. Analysts should also investigate the metabolism of the drug(s) of interest to help identify the drug and (or) its metabolite(s). Even after all precautions have been taken, one cannot rely completely on any screening test for drugs without using not only one's experience but also a confirmatory test to back up the primary screening test.

Note: Evaluators T.W.F. and L.P. also affirm the need to be familiar with the metabolite pattern of the drugs investigated and the potential for many drugs to give reactions to form colored spots and migrate in a manner that may cause them to be falsely identified as the drugs of interest. They suggest that virtually all drugs should be confirmed by alternative methods.

Sensitivity

Table 8 summarizes the sensitivity of the method for drugs routinely detected and reported. The sensitivity of detection of barbiturates can be increased by extracting urine with chloroform/isobutanol at an acidic pH (e.g., pH 2.0). The extraction of meprobamate and glutethimide, both neutral drugs, is essentially independent of pH. The pH of the extraction used here has been adjusted to optimize extraction of morphine; isobutanol is included in the extraction solvent for the same reason. Increasing the concentration of isobutanol will give some increase in sensitivity to morphine concentration, but the time to evaporate the solvent completely also increases.

Specimen Stability

When testing for the presence of drugs of abuse in urine specimens, the stability of the drugs is often questioned, especially when several days elapse between collection and receipt of specimens. Some forensic situations may require that urine specimens be saved for weeks after drugs of abuse have been determined. Frings and Queen (5) report that urine specimens stored for 14 days without refrigeration or preservatives remain suitable for qualitative tests for morphine, codeine, quinine, methadone, cocaine, barbiturates, and amphetamines. The storage conditions they studied were: room temperature (about 24 °C), with and without sodium azide (1 g/L); 37 (±1) °C, with and without sodium azide; and frozen (−20 °C). Other studies (4) have shown that

Table 8. Minimum Detection Limits of Selected Drugs

	Concn, mg/L		Concn, mg/L
Amitriptyline	1	Methadone	1
Amphetamine	2	Methamphetamine	0.5
Cocaine (as benzoylecgonine)	4	Morphine	0.5
		Nortriptyline	1
Codeine	0.5	Phencyclidine	1
Desipramine	1	Phenmetrazine	2
Doxepin	1	Phenobarbital	1
Glutethimide	1	Phenylpropanolamine	4
Hydromorphone	1	Propoxyphene	1
Imipramine	1	Pseudoephedrine	5
Meperidine	2	Secobarbital	0.5
Meprobamate	2		

salicylates, glutethimide, and meprobamate are stable in urine for six months when stored at 4 to 7 °C.

This method offers the analyst the capability of screening for drugs of abuse in a large number of urine specimens. The behavior (migration and color characteristics) of more than 85 drugs in this system is summarized here. The method is easy to set up and perform, involves readily obtainable reagents, requires no sophisticated instrumentation, and offers the sensitivity and specificity necessary for such a screening method. The procedure has been used in the Submitter's laboratory for many years, and more than 400 000 specimens have been analyzed without any major difficulties.

References

1. Davidow B, LiPetri N, Quame B. A thin layer chromatographic screening procedure for detecting drug abuse. *Am J Clin Pathol* **50**, 714-719 (1968).
2. Owen P, Pendlebury A, Moffat AC. Choice of thin-layer chromatographic systems for the routine screening for neutral drugs during toxicological analysis. *J Chromatogr* **161**, 187-193 (1978).
3. Owen P, Pendlebury A, Moffat AC. Choice of thin-layer chromatographic systems for the routine screening for acidic drugs during toxicological analysis. *J Chromatogr* **161**, 195-203 (1978).
4. Frings CS. Drug screening. *Crit Rev Clin Lab Sci* **4**, 357-382 (1973).
5. Frings CS, Queen CA. Stability of certain drugs of abuse in urine specimens. *Clin Chem* **18**, 1442 (1972). Letter.

Screening Procedures. II. Multiple Drugs by Gas-Liquid Chromatography

Submitters: Francis Avery Ragan, Jr., Stephen A. Hite, and Victoria R. Giblin, *Departments of Pathology, LSU Medical Center and Charity Hospital, New Orleans, LA 70112*

Evaluator: William D. Hemphill, *Hunt Laboratory, Inc., Metairie, LA 70002*

Introduction

In a case of suspected drug overdose, it is desirable to be able to screen rapidly for the more common drugs of abuse. Because of its speed, separation efficiency, and quantitative capacity, gas-liquid chromatography (GLC) is an excellent technique for drug analysis.

To be used to its fullest advantage, gas-liquid chromatography requires a rapid and sensitive method of sample preparation that provides a relatively clean extract for chromatography. The charcoal extraction method of Meola and Vanko (1,2), evaluated thoroughly by Adams (3) and described in detail by Gudzinowicz and Gudzinowicz (4), produces samples with a low background and has the advantage of being faster than methods involving XAD-2, ionic SA-2 resin, or Florisil as the extraction medium.

Principle

Drugs in biological material are extracted with charcoal, eluted from the charcoal by a mixture of organic solvents, concentrated in the eluate, and injected onto the gas-chromatographic column. The compounds are identified by comparing their retention times, relative to an internal standard, with the relative retention times of pure standards. The identification is then confirmed by an alternative method if possible.

Materials and Methods

Reagents

1. *Activated charcoal:* Norit A (J. T. Baker Chemical Co., Phillipsburg, NJ 08865).
2. *De-ionized water:* at least chromatographic-grade.
3. *Mixed extraction solvent:* Methylene chloride/isopropanol/diethyl ether (65/10/25, by vol), distilled in glass (Burdick and Jackson Laboratories, Inc., Muskegon, MI).
4. *Carbonate buffer, pH 11:* Sodium carbonate (Na_2CO_3), AR grade (Mallinckrodt Chemical Works, St. Louis, MO 63160). Dissolve 21 g in de-ionized water, then dilute to 2 L and adjust to pH 11.
5. *Barbital stock solution, 1 g/L:* Place 50 mg of sodium barbital (purified, J. T. Baker Chemical Co.) in a 50-mL volumetric flask and add de-ionized water to volume.

    Note: The solution is stable for one year under refrigeration.

6. *Barbital working solution, 40 mg/L:* Dilute 4 mL of stock barbital solution to 100 mL with de-ionized water.

Apparatus

1. *Gas chromatograph* with flame-ionization detectors, equipped for either capillary or packed columns. We used a Series 5710 gas chromatograph (Hewlett-Packard, Avondale, PA 19311) equipped with either a standard packed-column injection port or an SGE Unijector in split mode (Scientific Glass Engineering, Inc., Austin, TX 78759) and a flame-ionization detector.
2. *OV-101 methyl silicone fused-silica capillary column:* an 0.52-µm-thick film-coated 12.5 m × 0.31 to 0.32 mm (i.d.) column, Carbowax deactivated (Hewlett-Packard).
3. *OV-17 µ-Partisorb bonded-phase column* (low load): 6 ft. (1.8 m) × 2 mm (i.d.) (Whatman, Inc., Clifton, NJ 07014).

Procedures

Serum or plasma

1. Transfer 1.0 mL of serum or plasma to a 15-mL glass-stoppered centrifuge tube.
2. Add 4 mg of charcoal, 1 mL of the 40 mg/L barbital internal standard, and 4 mL of de-ionized water to the tube and stopper the tube.

    Note: After an initial measurement, the amount of charcoal may be estimated for future samples.

3. Vortex-mix the tube's contents vigorously for 30 s.
4. Centrifuge the tube for 2 min at $1000 \times g$. The charcoal should form a hard button in the bottom of the tube.
5. Decant the liquid and, keeping the tube inverted, tap the tube on an absorbant surface to remove as much liquid as possible.
6. Vortex-mix to disperse the charcoal over the inner surface of the tube. (Otherwise, the recovery of the extracted drugs will be lowered.)
7. Add 0.5 mL of the mixed extraction solvent to the tube and stopper.
8. Repeat steps 3 and 4.
9. Decant the solvent carefully into a clean stoppered tube. Do not transfer any of the remaining aqueous phase.
10. Evaporate the solvent to approximately 30 µL (not dryness) under a gentle stream of nitrogen.

    Note: Taking the sample to dryness will affect recovery unless the sample is reconstituted properly, by adding 0.5 mL of solvent, and heating briefly in a water bath, vortex-mixing vigorously, then evaporating to 30 µL as before.

11. Inject the sample (1 µL for the capillary column and 3 µL for packed columns) into the gas chromatograph and start the temperature program (see below).

Urine

1. Transfer 5 mL of urine to a 15-mL glass-stoppered centrifuge tube.

2. Add 4 mg of charcoal and 250 μL of stock barbital internal standard to the tube.

Note: The charcoal may be estimated after the initial measurement.

3. Vortex-mix 30 s, add 1 mL of pH 11 carbonate buffer, then vortex-mix again for 30 s.

4. Proceed with steps 4 through 11 for serum samples.

Gastric fluids

1. Transfer 1 mL of filtered gastric contents to a 15-mL glass-stoppered centrifuge tube.

2. Add 25 mg of charcoal, 250 μL of stock barbital internal standard, and 4 mL of de-ionized water.

Note: The charcoal may be estimated after the initial measurement.

3. Vortex-mix 30 s, then add 1 mL of pH 11 carbonate buffer and vortex-mix again for 30 s.

Note: This sequence must be followed exactly to ensure maximum recovery of barbiturates.

4. Check the pH of the mixture; if not alkaline, add additional carbonate buffer and vortex-mix for 30 s.

5. Proceed with steps 4 through 11 for serum samples.

Instrument Conditions

For the OV-101 column use the following settings: carrier gas, helium; flow rate, 1.75 mL/min (linear velocity, 38.5 cm/s); split ratio, 1:1: injector temperature, 250 °C; detector, 300 °C; oven, programmed from 120 to 250 °C at 16 °C/min, then a 4-min hold at 250 °C.

For the OV-17 column the carrier gas is also helium, and the head pressure is 414 kPa (60 psi), to give a flow rate of 41 mL/min. The injector temperature is 250 °C, the detector temperature is 300 °C, and the oven is programmed from 130 to 280 °C at 16 °C/min with an 8-min hold at 280 °C.

Calculations

To identify an unknown peak, determine its relative retention time and compare it with the relative retention time of a standard. Measure the distance in millimeters from the solvent front to the peak of the unknown and divide this by the distance from the solvent front to the peak of the internal standard. This number must be compared with relative retention times of standards obtained under the same conditions as that for the unknown. The use of relative retention times eliminates some of the variability inherent in gas chromatography. (See Appendix A for a list of relative retention times from various systems in the Submitters' laboratory.)

Discussion and Comments

The method described above for the analysis of drugs in physiological fluids is rapid and very easy to use in any clinical laboratory with a minimum of equipment, but several precautions should be taken. A sample may be extracted and prepared for injection in approximately 10 min and chromatographed in an additional 12 min. Samples may be injected about every 15 min, including column equilibration time, if prepared in batches.

The relative retention times reported in this procedure (e.g., Table 1) will vary from system to system and must be verified by the use of standards. This will correct for such variables as the flow rate of the carrier gas, column size, percent loading or thickness of the stationary phase, and variations of the flow rate and temperature during programming of the chromatographic oven. Tables of relative retention times should be developed for each system, and each time a drug is detected, the relative retention time should be recorded so that a retention window can be developed for each drug. The retention times listed in Appendix A provide a guide for approximate retention times while the user is developing his or her own index.

Table 1. Relative Retention Times of Some Drugs with the Columns Described Here

Drug	Relative retention time[a]	
	OV-101	OV-17
Methyprylon	0.87	1.09
Amobarbital	1.39	1.29
Meprobamate	1.59	1.55
Phenobarbital	2.01	1.76
Methaqualone	2.05	2.08
Diazepam	2.61	2.69
Phenytoin	2.86	2.55

[a]Relative to barbital = 1.00.

More than 160 drugs, metabolites, and interfering substances have been extracted by this system in our laboratory. Although recoveries vary, our experience is that the sensitivity of the method is similar to that of thin-layer chromatographic procedures (approximately 0.5 to 2 mg/L). However, this method is designed for analysis of specimens in overdose situations, not for detection of substance abuse.

Note: Phencyclidine has been quantified in the Submitters' laboratory in the high ng/L range and is run daily at 5 μg/L.

The analytical recovery of drugs in the charcoal extraction varies from about 25 to 75% for drug concentrations of 20 mg/L (3). This percentage is highly variable in a specimen containing multiple drugs, and one drug in the mixture may be preferentially extracted. However, this does not present a problem in analyzing a specimen containing multiple drugs unless quantification is desired.

Note: Evaluator W. D. H. reported recoveries of barbiturates from less than 10% to 42%.

Chromatographing some drugs (e.g., meprobamate) presents problems because they are degraded in the injection port, which decreases sensitivity and results in poor peak shape. This problem also occurs with such drugs as phenobarbital, acetaminophen, and diazepam (see Appendix A). Some drugs, such as Artane (trihexyphenidyl HCl) and flurazepam, are ordinarily not detected; often, only their metabolites will be detected in the specimen.

Controls should be run daily. The relative retention times should be recorded and peak shape evaluated to determine the condition of the chromatographic system. Controls may be obtained from a commercial source or prepared in-house. The control whose components are reported in Table 1 (Ortho Toxicology Control; Ortho Diagnostic Systems, Inc., Raritan, NJ 08869) combines both early- and late-eluting compounds, thermally labile compounds such as meprobamate, acidic barbiturates, and a poorly extracted barbiturate such as phenobarbital. This combination makes it a good control for evaluating the chromatographic system.

References

1. Meola J, Vanko M. A simple system for drug analysis. *Clin Chem* **17**, 637 (1971). Abstract.
2. Meola J, Vanko M. The use of charcoal in qualitative and quantitative analysis of drugs. *Clin Chem* **18**, 713 (1972). Abstract.
3. Adams RF. Drug analysis by simultaneous dual-column GLC Part 1: Very rapid clinical screening for restricted drugs in serum. *Clin Chem Newsl* **4**, 15 (1972). A publication of Perkin-Elmer, Norwalk, CT.
4. Gudzinowicz BJ, Gudzinowicz MJ. Drug isolation from biological media. In *Analysis of Drugs and Metabolites by Gas Chromatography-Mass Spectrometry*, **2**, Marcel Dekker, Inc., New York, NY, 1977, pp 69-82.

Appendix A: Characterization of Various Drugs by the Described Gas-Liquid Chromatographic Procedure with Use of Several Columns

The following listings are intended as guidelines only. Some, but not all, metabolites for a given drug may be listed. Some retention times listed are averages from many samples of commonly encountered drugs; others are for drugs seen only rarely. Each drug will have its own retention time "window," which has to be characterized for the individual chromatograph. Likewise, the impurities on each system must be characterized: many are seen, but not all are listed here.

The MS-II is a new system in the Submitters' laboratory; retention times for many drugs are still being tabulated.

A dash indicates that injection of a standard gave no response under these conditions.

Drug	Relative retention time[a] Capillary column	Relative retention time[a] Packed column	Absolute retention time, min MS I column	Absolute retention time, min MS II column
Acetaminophen[b,c]	1.622	1.48	6.3	5.4
Amitriptyline	2.155	1.99	7.9	8.8
Metab I[d]	1.749	1.69	6.1	7.3
Metab II	2.157	2.06	7.5	
Metab III	2.339	2.29	10.1	
Metab IV	2.438	2.62	11.1	
Metab V	2.578	2.46		
Amobarbital	1.392	1.29	4.9	
Metab I	1.965	1.64	6.6	
Metab II	1.425	1.39	4.9	
Metab III	2.288	1.92	7.3	
Amphetamine	0.236	0.34	1.2	
Atropine		2.05		
Barbital	1.000	1.00	3.4	3.9
Benzphetamine	1.435	1.43	5.2	
Benztropine	2.272			
Brompheniramine	1.993	1.82	6.9	
Butabarbital	1.256	1.25	4.4	5.2
Butalbital	1.305	1.23	4.5	
Caffeine	1.380	1.60	5.1	6.1
Camphor				
Peak I[e]		0.31		
Peak II		0.74		
Carbamazepine[f]	2.291	1.90	8.2	9.3
Metab I		7.1	8.3	
Thermal product I			5.9	7.3
Thermal product II	1.813	1.92	6.6	7.7
Thermal product III			4.9	6.0
Carbromal	0.852	degrades	3.2	
Peak I	0.289	0.49	1.5	
Peak II	0.520		2.2	
Carisoprodol	1.577	1.42	5.6	
Chlordiazepoxide	2.625	3.10	10.2	
Chlormezanone	2.179		7.7	
Peak II	0.290	0.48	1.5	
Peak III			7.1	
Chlorpheniramine	1.776	1.71	6.3	
Chlorpromazine	2.646	2.64	9.2	
Metab I	2.178	2.20	8.0	
Metab II	2.225	2.27	7.8	
Metab III	2.719			
Chlorpropamide	1.525	1.52	4.8	5.4
Metab I	0.753	1.17	3.1	
Cocaine	2.128	2.10	7.4	8.7
Codeine	2.480	2.52	8.6	9.9
Cyclobenzaprine	2.189	2.03	7.8	
Cyproheptadine	2.490			
Desipramine	2.205	2.13	6.0	
Desmethyldiazepam	2.728	3.05	9.5	
Diethylpropion				
Peak I	0.873	0.95	3.0	
Peak II	0.739	0.86	—	
Diazepam[b]	2.610	2.69	8.7	10.4
Dihydrocodeine	2.600	—	—	
Diphenhydramine	1.508	1.51	5.4	6.6
Metab I	—	1.55	—	
Doxepin	2.160	2.03	7.6	
Metab I	2.034	1.75	7.5	
Metab II	2.182	2.10		
Metab III	2.408			
Metab IV	2.427			
Metab V	2.497			
Metab VI	1.618	—	5.7	
Doxylamine	1.622	1.61	5.7	7.0
Metab I			4.0	
Metab II			3.5	4.4
Metab III	2.230	2.22	8.0	9.1
Metab IV	2.322	2.31	8.3	9.4
Ephedrine				
Peak I	0.544	0.71	2.2	
Peak II	0.483	0.69		
Ethchlorvynol	0.203	0.30	1.1	
Ethinamate	0.606	0.80	2.3	
Ethosuximide	0.361	0.55	1.6	
Fenoprofen	1.536	1.64	6.5	
Flurazepam[f]	3.168	3.71	11.2	
Metab I	2.958			
Glutethimide	1.506	1.60	5.3	
Metab I	1.618	1.66	5.7	
Metab II	1.779	1.87	6.1	
Metab III		2.07		
Metab IV				2.31

Drug	Relative retention time[a] Capillary column	Relative retention time[a] Packed column	Absolute retention time, min MS I column	Absolute retention time, min MS II column
Homocaine (ecgonine ethyl ester benzoate)			7.8	9.0
Hydroxyzine	—	—	—	
Ibuprofen	1.102	1.06		
Imipramine	2.165	2.05	7.6	
Metab I (see Desipramine)				
Metab II	1.519	1.66	5.7	
Lidocaine	1.560	1.55	5.6	6.7
Metab I			5.0	6.2
Loxapine	2.893	2.85		
Metab I	2.966	3.13		
Metab II	3.094			
Maprotiline	2.358	2.25	8.3	
Meperidine	1.270	1.34	4.7	
Metab I	1.404			
Mephenoxalone			7.6	
Mephentermine	0.380	0.46	1.7	
Mephobarbital	1.597	1.62	5.7	
Meprobamate	1.590	1.55	5.5	6.0
Thermal product	0.733	0.93	3.0	3.1
Methadone	2.063	1.89	7.1	
Metab I	1.866	1.73	6.4	
Metab II			7.3	8.4
Methamphetamine	0.298	0.39	1.3	
Methapyrilene	2.659	1.73	6.2	
Methaqualone	2.048	2.08	7.2	
Metab I	2.497	2.71	9.5	
Metab II	2.839			
Metab III	2.723			
d-Methorphan	1.993	1.92	7.1	8.5
Methylphenidate	1.157		4.4	
Methyprylon	0.873	1.09	3.3	
Metab I	0.937	1.14		
Metab II	0.948			
Molindone	1.649	1.71	5.8	
Morphine	2.517	2.74	8.9	
Naloxone	3.074	—	—	
Nicotine	0.478	0.67	2.1	2.9
Metab I	1.160	1.47	4.2	5.3
Metab II				5.9
Nitrazepam	3.732	4.74	12.0	
Orphenadrine	1.583	1.60		
Metab I		1.66		
Oxazepam	2.257	2.38	9.2	
Oxycodone	2.740	2.98	9.1	
PCH	0.455		3.1	
PEMA	1.707	1.75	6.0	
Pentazocine	2.354	2.11	7.9	
Pentobarbital	1.406	1.34	5.1	
Phenacetin	1.207	1.37	4.6	
Phencyclidine (PCP)	1.571	1.48	5.7	
Phendimetrazine	0.734	0.85	2.8	
Pheniramine	1.400	1.40	5.0	
Phenmetrazine	0.668	0.80	2.6	
Phenobarbital[c]	2.013	1.76	6.6	7.3
Phentermine	0.262	0.36	1.7	
Metab I	0.178			
Phenylbutazone			9.1	
Phenytoin[c]	2.855	2.55	8.6	9.5
Metab I			7.7	8.8
Phenylpropanolamine	0.474	0.70	2.0	
Phthalate no. 1	1.149	1.11	2.2	
Phthalate no. 2	1.356	1.58	6.4	7.0
Phthalate no. 3	1.607	2.66	3.4	
Phthalate no. 4			9.0	
Primidone	2.422	2.53	8.0	
Procaine	0.822	1.82	6.5	
Propoxyphene	2.132	2.32	7.4	8.7
Metab I	2.507	2.37	8.4	10.0
Metab IIA	2.548	1.07	3.7	4.8
Metab IIB	2.572	1.27	4.3	5.4
Metab III	2.868	2.74	8.4	10.2
Metab IV			8.5	10.3
Metab V			7.4	
Metab VI				8.3
Propylhexedrine	0.267	0.27	1.3	
Protriptyline	—	—	—	
Pseudoephedrine	0.385	0.69	2.3	
Pyribenzamine	1.745	1.70	6.1	7.4
Pyrilamine	2.223.	2.11	7.6	
Quinine				
Peak I	3.776			
Peak II	3.826			
Secobarbital	1.497	1.42	5.3	6.1
Metab I		1.79	7.0	
Talbutal		1.31		
Theobromine		1.77	6.0	6.5
Theophylline[c]	1.875	1.88	7.0	6.7
Thiopental	1.636	1.51	5.6	
Thonzylamine	2.173			
Trihexyphenidyl[f]	2.239	2.05	7.7	
Metab I	2.670	2.61	9.1	
Trimipramine			7.6	8.8
Vacutainer Tube impurity	2.448	2.12	8.4	9.8

[a] Relative to the internal standard, barbital.
[b] Chromatographs poorly.
[c] Poor sensitivity.
[d] The numbering of metabolites (i.e., Metab I, Metab II, etc.) is the Submitters' own and does not correspond to any system cited in the literature.
[e] The source of compounds labeled Peak I, Peak II, etc. is uncertain. They may be metabolites, thermal degradation products, isomeric compounds, or some other form arising from the parent drug.
[f] Often, only metabolites are detected.

Screening Procedures. III. Basic Drugs in Urine

Submitters: Robert W. Dalrymple and Frank M. Stearns, *Damon Clinical Laboratories, Trevose, PA 19047*

Evaluator: Gerald E. Clement, *Lehigh Valley Hospital Center, Allentown, PA 18102*

Introduction

Toxicology laboratories frequently screen urine samples of suspected overdose patients. Often, these "stat" requests are drug-specific, being based on clinical evaluation and the patient's history.

Highly specific and sensitive procedures such as thin-layer chromatography *(1-3)*, gas chromatography *(4,5)*, mass spectrometry *(6-8)*, and gas chromatography-mass spectrometry *(9-11)* are used for drug detection, but are time consuming and require expensive instruments or a high level of expertise. Immunoassay methods, specifically the EMIT™ system (Syva Co., Palo Alto, CA) *(12)*, have become quite popular by providing quick results with acceptable sensitivity at minimal cost. However, drug detection by this technique is limited to the number of drug-specific kits available from the manufacturer.

Several rapid and inexpensive spot tests are available for simplified detection of phenothiazines *(13)*, amitriptyline *(14)*, imipramine *(15)*, chlordiazepoxide *(16)*, meprobamate *(17)*, ethchlorvynol *(18)*, salicylate *(19)*, and halogenated hydrocarbons *(20)*, and are currently in wide use.

Recently, a simple color test has been developed in which tetrabromophenolphthalein ethyl ester (TBP) in chloroform is used for detecting basic drugs in urine. Originally described by Saker and Solomons *(21)* as a rapid presumptive test for phencyclidine and other cross-reacting substances in urine, this work was subsequently expanded by Rio and Hodnett *(22)* to include more than 60 drugs, demonstrating the broad specificity of the test. The publication by Rio and Hodnett also included a compilation of the sensitivity limits of the TBP reagent. The versatility of this rapid, broad-spectrum spot test has obvious utility in the emergency toxicology laboratory.

Principle

A urine aliquot is buffered to pH 6-7 with use of a pH 7.0 buffer concentrate. TBP in chloroform is added and the sample is vortex-mixed. The development of color in the lower chloroform layer, if greater than that of a drug-free urine, is recorded as a positive test result.

Materials and Methods

Equipment

1. 10 × 75 mm disposable culture tubes (cat. no. 14-962-10A; Fisher Scientific Co., Pittsburgh, PA).
2. Jumbo pipette bulbs (cat. no. 13-711-7; Fisher Scientific Co.).
3. Vortex-type mixer.

Reagents

1. pH 7.0 buffer concentrate. Transfer 68 g of KH_2PO_4 (cat. no. P-284; Fisher Scientific Co.) to a 500-mL volumetric flask. Dissolve in about 450 mL of distilled water. Adjust to pH 7.0 with NaOH (6 mol/L), then dilute to volume with distilled water. Stable for one year at 2-7 °C.

2. Chloroform (cat. no. C-298; Fisher Scientific Co.).

3. Sulfuric acid, 1.8 mol/L. To 80 mL of distilled water in a 100-mL volumetric flask add 10.8 mL of concentrated sulfuric acid. Mix thoroughly, cool, and dilute to volume with distilled water. Stable for at least one year at room temperature.

4. TBP reagent. Dissolve 50 mg of tetrabromophenolphthalein ethyl ester (cat. no. 6810; Fisher Scientific Co.) in 100 mL of chloroform in a 100-mL volumetric flask. Add 1.0 mL of the H_2SO_4 solution, and shake for 2 to 3 min. Aspirate the aqueous phase. Stable for three months stored at 2-7 °C in a brown glass bottle.

> *Evaluator G.E.C.:* The reagents are very stable and, in our experience, we have never observed that the reagents go "bad."

Controls

1. Negative control. Pooled drug-free urine.

2. Positive control. Prepare the positive control for the drug of interest by utilizing the established sensitivity limit listed in Table 1. For example: Phencyclidine positive control, 0.5 mg/L. Weigh 14.5 mg of phencyclidine HCl and transfer to a 25-mL flask. Dissolve and dilute to volume with methanol. Transfer 500 µL of this stock to a 500-mL volumetric flask. Dilute to volume with drug-free urine and mix thoroughly. Frozen aliquots are stable for up to 12 months.

Specimen

Collect 50 mL of random (untimed) urine; refrigerate if screening will be delayed. Retain sufficient volume to confirm positive results with an alternative technique.

Procedure

1. Place 2 mL of controls and unknowns in 10 × 75 mm tubes.
2. Add three drops of the pH 7.0 buffer concentrate; vortex-mix.

Table 1. Drug Sensitivities with the TBP Color Reagent: Minimum Concentrations Distinguishable from Drug-Free Urine

Drug	Concn, mg/L	Drug	Concn, mg/L	Drug	Concn, mg/L
Acetophenazine	2.0	Flurazepam	2.0	Phendimetrazine	5.0
Adiphenine	2.0	Haloperidol	5.0	Phenethylamine	>10.0
Aminopyrine	>10.0	Hydrocodone	2.0	Phenindamine	2.0
Amitriptyline	1.0	Hydromorphone	>10.0	Pheniramine	1.0
Amoxapine	5.0	Hydroxyzine	>10.0	Phenmetrazine	5.0
Amphetamine	>10.0	Hyoscyamine	1.0	Phenyltoloxamine	2.0
Antazoline	1.0	Imipramine	1.0	Physostigmine	1.0
Benactyzine	2.0	Levallorphan	1.0	Pipamazine	2.0
Benzphetamine	2.0	Loxapine	5.0	Piperocaine	1.0
Benzthiazide	>10.0	Maprotiline	1.0	Prilocaine	>10.0
Benztropine	1.0	Meclizine	5.0	Procainamide	10.0
Bromodiphenhydramine	1.0	Meperidine	2.0	Procaine	2.0
Brompheniramine	1.0	Mephentermine	2.0	Prochlorperazine	2.0
Buclizine	5.0	Mepivacaine	1.0	Procyclidine	1.0
Carbetapentane	1.0	Mesoridazine	2.0	Promethazine	1.0
Carbinoxamine	1.0	Metabutoxycaine	1.0	Propiomazine	1.0
Carisoprodol	5.0	Methadone	0.5	Propoxyphene	2.0
Carphenazine	2.0	EDDP metabolite[a]	0.5	Propranolol	1.0
Chlorcyclizine	1.0	EMDP metabolite[b]	0.5	Propylhexedrine	1.0
Chlorothen	1.0	Methamphetamine	5.0	Prothipendyl	1.0
Chlorpheniramine	1.0	Methaphenilene	1.0	Protriptyline	1.0
Chlorpromazine	2.0	Methapyrilene	1.0	Pyrilamine	1.0
Chlorprothixene	>10.0	Methdilazine	1.0	Quinacrine	1.0
Clemizole	1.0	Methixene	1.0	Quinidine	1.0
Clomipramine	1.0	Methoxyphenamine	1.0	Quinine	1.0
Codeine	2.0	Methoxypromazine	1.0	Scopolamine	>10.0
Cyclizine	1.0	Methylphenidate	1.0	Strychnine	2.0
Desipramine	2.0	Naphazoline	1.0	Tetracaine	2.0
Dextromethorphan	2.0	Neostigmine	>10.0	Thenyldiamine	1.0
Diethylpropion	2.0	Nicotine	>10.0	Thiethylperazine	2.0
Dihydrocodeine	2.0	Nordoxepin	2.0	Thioridazine	2.0
Diphenhydramine	2.0	Norpropoxyphene	2.0	Thiothixene	5.0
Diphenylpyraline	1.0	Nylidrin	2.0	Thonzylamine	1.0
Doxepin	1.0	Orphenadrine	1.0	Trifluoperazine	5.0
Doxylamine	2.0	Papaverine	5.0	Triflupromazine	2.0
Ephedrine	>10.0	Pargyline	>10.0	Trimeprazine	2.0
Ethopropazine	1.0	Pentazocine	1.0	Trimethobenzamide	5.0
Ethylmorphine	2.0	Perphenazine	>10.0	Trimipramine	1.0
Fenfluramine	1.0	Phenacaine	1.0	Tripelennamine	1.0
Fluphenazine	5.0	Phencyclidine	0.5	Triprolidine	1.0

[a] 2-Ethylidene-1,5-dimethyl-3,3-diphenylpyrrolidine. [b] 2-Ethyl-5-methyl-3,3-diphenylpyrroline.

3. Add 0.2 mL of TBP reagent to each tube.
4. Vortex-mix 10 s.
5. After letting the sample stand 5 min, record as positive the development of any color in the TBP/chloroform layer that is greater than that of the drug-free urine control.

Discussion

Basic drugs form various colored complexes with the TBP reagent. These complexes, which are stable for several hours, range from a light yellow-brown or orange to amethyst or deep blue. The specific color developed depends on the particular substance present and its concentration. Although color data for a number of drugs have been published (22) to aid identification, relying on these data is unwise and not recommended. At the minimum sensitivities listed in Table 1, most substances react with TBP to give a light brown color. Any positive or marginally positive result must be confirmed by an alternative drug-specific technique such as EMIT or chromatography.

Evaluator G.E.C.: The color development is all important. Almost all drugs produce a brown-red color that can be suggestive of a positive test. We have found yellows, light orange, and light green colors to be negative for no drugs identified.

The Submitters have reviewed and expanded the work by Rio and Hodnett (22) and others to list more than 100

Table 2. Drugs Found Not to React with the TBP Color Reagent at 1000 mg/L

Acetaminophen	Disulfiram	Methyprylon	Phenylpropanolamine
Acetazolamide	Ethchlorvynol	Mescaline	Primidone
Benzoylecgonine	Ethinamate	Morphine	Salicylate
Caffeine	Glutethimide	Nordiazepam	Secobarbital
Carbamazepine	4-Hydroxyglutethimide	Oxycodone	Theophylline
Chlordiazepoxide	Indomethacin	Oxymorphone	Tolbutamide
Cocaine	Isoniazid	Phenacetin	Tranylcypromine
Diazepam	Lidocaine	Phenylbutazone	Trazodone
Diflunisal	Meprobamate	Phenylephrine	

drugs that react positively with the TBP reagent. The sensitivity limits for these substances are listed in Table 1. Additionally, we have identified 35 drugs that do not react at concentrations of up to 1000 mg/mL; these are listed in Table 2.

The precise mechanism for the color formation between TBP and basic drugs has not been thoroughly investigated. The reaction apparently depends on the ability of a nitrogen atom to donate its unshared electron pair to the electrophilic TBP structure. Substances with an aromatic ring that is one to three carbons removed from a secondary or tertiary amine show the greatest sensitivity. The CH_2 groups act as insulators and prevent the transfer of electronic charge from the amine to the aromatic ring; therefore, the electron density on the amine group remains high. Conversely, substances with a carboxyl or aromatic ring adjacent to the amine, and substances with structures that provide a mechanism for dispersion of the amine group's electron density, fail to react with the TBP reagent.

False positives from endogenous, nondrug constituents in urine have not been observed, nor is there documented evidence of a positive TBP reaction related to trauma or hormonal processes. Caffeine and nicotine, which are frequently found in urine, react minimally with the TBP reagent and do not interfere. However, the Submitters have found that the TBP reagent will darken slightly when added to drug-free urine samples that have been held at room temperature for more than 72 h. If the screening with TBP must be delayed, we recommend that the urine samples be stored at 2-7 °C.

As previously noted (21), this test has little value in screening urine samples from patients on maintenance therapy. TBP can detect methadone at 0.5 mg/mL and will consistently give positive results for individuals receiving this medication.

Negative results for TBP screens may suggest the absence of those drugs listed in Table 1. However, further testing with more sophisticated and sensitive techniques is certainly indicated when the urine sample is from a comatose patient. Several basic compounds do not give a positive reaction with TBP—including cocaine and its metabolite benzoylecgonine, several opiates including morphine, and two frequently abused benzodiazepines, diazepam and chlordiazepoxide.

Clinical Illustrations

The procedure has been successfully used by the Submitters in two other areas. First, the reagent has considerable utility in screening gastric fluids of suspected overdose patients. Because ingested substances are often found in higher concentrations in gastric samples, all the drugs listed in Table 1 may be detected. Two cases illustrate the usefulness of the TBP screen:

Case 1. A gastric sample of a suspected overdose patient was submitted to the laboratory for analysis. An aliquot was screened with the TBP reagent by the outlined procedure. The development of a deep reddish-purple color suggested the presence of one of the drugs listed in Table 1. Subsequent analysis of the sample by a dual-column gas-chromatographic technique (4) led to a positive identification of the drug as doxepin.

Case 2. Another gastric sample screened with the TBP reagent gave no color change, thus ruling out the drugs listed in Table 1. Attention was therefore focused on substances that do not react with TBP (Table 2). After further screening, the sample was reported as positive for acetaminophen.

The second area involves the identification of pills and other related substances for medico-legal purposes. Two more cases demonstrate this utility:

Case 3. A syringe with a dark liquid was submitted for analysis, with little ancillary information. When the solution was further diluted with water and tested with the TBP reagent, a deep purple color formed in the lower chloroform layer. Further analysis for basic drugs by chromatography identified the drug as fenfluramine.

Case 4. Pill samples were submitted to the laboratory for identification. The pills were crushed and 2 to 3 mg of the powder was tested with the TBP reagent. No coloration was observed and the basic drugs from Table 1 were eliminated from consideration. This pill was identified as phenylbutazone by a gas-chromatographic procedure with confirmation by ultraviolet spectroscopy.

In conclusion, the TBP screening procedure is rapid, simple to perform, and inexpensive, and provides acceptable sensitivity for a large number of basic drugs that may be involved in overdose situations. The test is useful in the emergency toxicology laboratory when used in conjunction with clinical evaluation and other sophisticated screening techniques.

Evaluator's Comments

In my laboratory, these tests have been extremely valuable, timely, and cost effective. We screen all urines and gastric specimens as part of our emergency toxicology protocol with this TBP reagent.

A positive color development is useful, but the Submitters should emphasize how important a *negative* test result can be. A negative result allows us to rule out a large number of basic drugs that do not contribute to diagnosing a comatose patient.

With experience, we have become very proficient in recognizing the red color development from tricyclic antidepressants. In our area, antidepressant drugs are widely prescribed, and thus lead to abuse and overdosing by patients. Fully 25% of our emergency requests suggest an antidepressant drug involvement. We, as do most other laboratories, quantify tricyclic antidepressants by liquid chromatography.

Because we can do only so many tests or quantifications within our 2-h turnaround time, a negative TBP result immediately allows us to rule out high concentrations of antidepressants and turn our testing to other classes of drugs. A negative urine result can be *immediately reported* to the physician as negative for antidepressants, which is clinically significant toxicology information.

We screen all routine drug requests with the TBP reagent. A positive urine TBP test result causes us to look even more closely at our thin-layer chromatographic screen of that patient.

We screen all our urine and gastric forensic specimens with the TBP test. A negative TBP result reassures us that we have not missed an important basic drug, whereas a positive result causes us to look more closely and expand our scope of testing.

During these days of severe cost-containment strategies, we have found the TBP test to be an extremely *clinically useful and cost-effective test*. This 10¢ test often is substituted for a $5 thin-layer chromatographic test in our laboratory.

References

1. Davidow B, Petri NL, Quame B. A thin-layer chromatographic screening procedure for detecting drug abuse. *Am J Clin Pathol* **50**, 714-719 (1968).
2. Mule SJ. Identification of narcotics, barbiturates, amphetamines, tranquilizers, and psychomimetics in human urine. *J Chromatogr* **39**, 202-311 (1969).
3. Kaistha KK, Jaffe JH. TLC techniques for identification of narcotics, barbiturates, and CNS stimulants in a drug abuse urine screening program. *J Pharm Sci* **61**, 679-689 (1972).
4. Foerster EH, Hatchett D, Garriott JC. A rapid, comprehensive screening procedure for basic drugs in blood or tissues by gas chromatography. *J Anal Toxicol* **2**, 50-55 (1978).
5. Ferslew KE, Manno BR, Manno JE. A rapid, semiautomated gas chromatographic system for the qualitative confirmation of selected drugs of abuse and metabolites from urine. *J Anal Toxicol* **3**, 30-34 (1979).
6. Foltz RL, Clarke PA, Knowlton DA, Hoyland JR. *The Rapid Identification of Drugs from Mass Spectra*, Batelle Laboratories, Columbus, OH, 1974.
7. Saferstein R, Manura JJ, De PK. Drug detection in urine by chemical ionization mass spectrometry. *J Forens Sci* **28**, 29-36 (1978).
8. Saferstein R, Manura JJ, Brettel TA, De PK. Drug detection in urine by chemical ionization mass spectrometry II. *J Anal Toxicol* **2**, 245-249 (1978).
9. Costello CE, Hertz HS, Sakai T, Bieman K. Routine use of a flexible gas chromatograph-mass spectrometer-computer system to identify drugs and their metabolites in body fluids of overdose victims. *Clin Chem* **20**, 255-265 (1974).
10. Finkle BS, Foltz RL, Taylor DM. A comprehensive GC-MS reference data system for toxicological and biomedical purposes. *J Chromatogr Sci* **12**, 304-328 (1974).
11. Ullucci PA, Cadoret R, Stasiowski PD, Martin HF. A comprehensive GC/MS drug screening procedure. *J Anal Toxicol* **2**, 33-38 (1978).
12. Bastiani RJ, Phillips RC, Schneider RS, Ullman EF. Homogeneous immunochemical drug assays. *Am J Med Technol* **39**, 211-216 (1973).
13. Forrest FM, Forrest IS, Mason AS. Review of rapid urine tests for phenothiazines and related drugs. *Am J Psychiatry* **118**, 300 (1961).
14. Decker WJ, Treuting J. Spot tests for rapid diagnosis of poisoning. *Clin Toxicol* **4**, 88 (1971).
15. Forrest IS, Forrest FM. A rapid urine color test for imipramine (Tofranil, Geigy). *Am J Psychiatry* **116**, 840 (1960).
16. *Products Reference Manual*, Roche Laboratories, Nutley, NJ, 1970.
17. Hoffman AJ, Ludwig BJ. An improved colorimetric method for the determination of meprobamate in biological fluids. *J Am Pharm Assoc* **48**, 740 (1959).
18. Frings CS, Cohen PS. Rapid colorimetric method for the quantitative determination of ethchlorvynol (Placidyl) in serum and urine. *Am J Clin Pathol* **54**, 833 (1970).
19. Keller WJ. A rapid method for the determination of salicylates in serum or plasma. *Am J Clin Pathol* **17**, 415 (1947).
20. Maehly AC. Volatile toxic compounds. *Prog Chem Toxicol* **3**, 68-79 (1967).
21. Saker EG. Solomons ET. A rapid and inexpensive presumptive test for phencyclidine and certain other cross-reacting substances. *J Anal Toxicol* **3**, 220-221 (1979).
22. Rio JG, Hodnett CN. Evaluation of a colormetric screening test for basic drugs in urine. *J Anal Toxicol* **5**, 267-269 (1981).

Screening Procedures. IV. Phenothiazines

Submitter: Christopher S. Frings, *Medical Laboratory Associates, Birmingham, AL 35256*

Evaluators: C. Ray Ratliff, *Bio-Analytic Laboratories, Inc., Palm City, FL 33490*

Ann Warner, *Institute de Medicina Forense, Universidad de Puerto Rico, San Juan, PR 00936*

Introduction

Phenothiazines are used in treating psychosis, but are also used for control of nausea and vomiting. Although phenothiazines have a high therapeutic index, they sometimes cause serious overdose.

Analysis of phenothiazines is complicated by the fact that many phenothiazine derivatives are used therapeutically and, further, that phenothiazines are extensively metabolized. Most quantitative methods for detecting phenothiazines in serum lack either sensitivity or specificity, and screening methods for phenothiazines lack specificity. The authors of the most widely used test for the qualitative detection of phenothiazines in urine, the "FPN" test, state: "the test produces immediate color reactions with the urines of patients who have ingested any phenothiazine compound, including the various antihistaminic compounds of this group" (1) and "the sensitive FPN test for the detection of urine phenothiazine compounds remains a valuable diagnostic tool, especially because of its absence of false negatives" (2).

This screening test for the qualitative detection of phenothiazines in urine is that of Forrest and Forrest (1,2).

Principle

Urine is mixed with a reagent ("FPN") containing ferric chloride, perchloric acid, and nitric acid. A chromogen (pink, purple, or blue) forms if certain phenothiazines are present.

Materials and Methods

FPN reagent. Mix 5 mL of freshly prepared $FeCl_3$ (50 g/L), 45 mL of perchloric acid (200 mL/L), and 50 mL of HNO_3 (500 mL/L). This reagent is stable for six months when stored in a brown bottle at room temperature.

Specimen handling. Urine samples are suitable for this assay for as long as one week stored at 4-7 °C or for at least one month when stored frozen. Serum or plasma samples are not satisfactory.

Procedure. Add 1 mL of FPN reagent to 1 mL of urine sample and mix. Note what color forms *immediately*—all colors appearing after 10 s must be disregarded. Depending upon which phenothiazine(s) and metabolites are present, the color may be pink, purple, or blue. If no color forms, report as none detected for phenothiazines. If a pink, purple, or blue color forms, report as positive for phenothiazines.

Discussion

Forrest and Forrest reported false-positive results with the FPN test with *p*-aminosalicylic acid, phenylpyruvic acid, high doses of estrogens, and urine from persons with impaired liver function. We emphasize that although some phenothiazines are detected by the FPN test at therapeutic concentrations, others—e.g., fluphenazine (Prolixin®)—are not. The test is not optimal as an indicator of whether a patient is taking certain prescribed phenothiazines, but does indicate gross overdosage for many of the phenothiazines.

References

1. Forrest IS, Forrest FM. Urine color test for the detection of phenothiazine compounds. *Clin Chem* **6,** 11-15 (1960).
2. Forrest IS, Forrest FM. Supplement to urine color test for the detection of phenothiazine compounds. *Clin Chem* **6,** 362-363 (1960).

Screening Procedures. V. Chlorinated Hydrocarbons

Submitters: Francis Avery Ragan, Jr., and Victoria R. Giblin, *Departments of Pathology, LSU Medical Center and Charity Hospital, New Orleans, LA 70112*

Evaluators: Joseph E. Manno, *Department of Pharmacology and Therapeutics, Toxicology Section, LSU Medical Center-Shreveport, Shreveport, LA 71130*
William D. Hemphill, *Hunt Laboratory, Inc., Metairie, LA 70006*

Introduction

This method for detecting chlorinated hydrocarbons is based on the Fujiwara reaction, which has undergone frequent minor modifications (1-4).

The Fujiwara reaction provides a rapid screening test for chlorinated hydrocarbons in laboratories not equipped for gas-liquid chromatographic analysis of volatile compounds in patients' specimens.

Compounds having from one to four chlorine atoms per molecule in the following classes are generally detected by the Fujiwara reaction: CCl_4, $CHCl_3$, CHR_2CCl_3, $CR_2(OH)CCl_3$, $RCHCl_2$, $CR_2=CRCl$, and $HRC=CHCl$.

Principle

The test is based on the reaction of halogenated hydrocarbons with sodium hydroxide in the presence of pyridine. In a positive reaction a pink to red color forms in the pyridine layer.

Materials and Methods

Reagents

1. *Pyridine, ACS reagent grade.* If not fresh, this should be distilled. Pyridine should be handled in a fume hood.

    Note: If pyridine is not freshly distilled, the sensitivity of the method will be decreased.

2. *Sodium hydroxide, ACS reagent grade.* Dissolve 10 g of sodium hydroxide in de-ionized water and dilute to 100 mL.

Collection and Handling of Specimens

Urine and gastric juice are the specimens of choice for this test. They should be collected as soon as possible after ingestion or exposure.

Procedure

1. Place 1 mL of sample (urine or gastric juice) in one tube and 1 mL of de-ionized water in a second tube for a blank.

    Note: Include the blank to check for contamination of the reagents by solvents commonly used in the laboratory.

2. Add 1 mL of NaOH solution to each tube.
3. Add 1 mL of pyridine to each tube.
4. Place the tubes in a water bath at 100 °C for 2 min.
5. Compare the tubes' contents. A pink to red color in the pyridine layer of the sample tube is positive. A color in the blank tube indicates contamination.

Discussion and Comments

The ingestion of chlorinated hydrocarbons presents a serious medical problem. The chlorinated hydrocarbons depress the central nervous system (CNS) and cause other pathological problems. The minimal lethal dose of carbon tetrachloride is 3-5 mL; this chemical causes severe hepatorenal problems after acute or chronic exposure, whereas chloroform is reportedly fatal (because of CNS depression) after ingestions of 10 mL (6). Dichloromethane, which is metabolized to carbon monoxide, produces anoxia as well as CNS depression. Trichloroethylene, which has been used as a solvent and an anesthetic agent, is metabolized to chloral hydrate and its metabolites. Chloral hydrate—a "Mickey Finn"—is metabolized to trichloroethanol and trichloroacetic acid (7). These are but a few of the chlorinated hydrocarbons on the market, and the assay results must be validated by analysis of an appropriate concentration of the suspected compound before being reported.

The Fujiwara reaction or one of its modifications is a rapid and sensitive method for screening patients' urine and gastric specimens for a chlorinated hydrocarbon. The method is most useful in situations where an acute exposure to a chlorinated hydrocarbon has been indicated by the patient's history and must be confirmed.

The Fujiwara reaction has been used to quantify trichloroethanol in serum or blood (4) and to differentiate chloral hydrate and chloroform in blood (2), but for such purposes head-space analysis by gas-liquid chromatography is preferred (5).

The sensitivity (least detectable concentration) of the Fujiwara method is reported to be 5 mg/L (2), but this will vary with the compound.

    Note: Evaluators J.E.M. and W.D.H. both reported the sensitivity of the method as 10 mg/L in urine.

Purity of the reagents is very important. The blank *must* be included in each run because the chlorinated solvents commonly used in a laboratory will contaminate the pyridine and interfere with the assay.

This method is not recommended for the determination of chronic exposure to chlorinated hydrocarbons. For that, a method such as head-space gas-liquid chromatography should be used.

References

1. Clarke EGC. *Isolation and Identification of Drugs*, Pharmaceutical Press, London, 1969, p 15.
2. Kaye S. *Handbook of Emergency Toxicology*, CC Thomas, Springfield, IL, 1970, pp 195-208.
3. Freimuth HC. Identification and estimation of volatile poisons. In *Toxicology, Mechanisms and Analytical Methods*, 2, CP Stewart, A Stolman, Eds., Academic Press, New York, NY, 1961, pp 75-77.
4. Friedman PJ, Cooper JR. Determination of chloral hydrate, trichloroacetic acid and trichloroethanol. *Anal Chem* 30, 1674 (1958).
5. Dubowski KM. Organic volatile substances. In *Methodology for Analytical Toxicology*, I Sunshine, Ed., CRC Press, Cleveland, OH, 1975, pp 407-411.
6. Baselt RC. *Disposition of Toxic Drugs and Chemicals in Man*, Biomedical Publishers, Canton, CT, 1978, pp 138-144.
7. Skoutakis VA. *Clinical Toxicology of Drugs*, Lea & Febiger, Philadelphia, PA, 1982, pp 89-90.

Acetaminophen by Liquid Chromatography

Submitters: William H. Porter, Linda D. Dorie, and Philip W. Rutter, *Department of Pathology, University of Kentucky Medical Center, Lexington, KY 40536*

Evaluators: Stephen W. Duckett and David C. Hohnadel, *Clinical Chemistry Laboratory, The Christ Hospital, Cincinnati, OH 45219*

E. Howard Taylor, *Department of Pathology, University of Arkansas for Medical Sciences, Little Rock, AR 72205*

Introduction

Acetaminophen, a widely used analgesic agent, causes significant hepatotoxicity in cases of overdose. Neither acetaminophen nor its major pharmacologically inactive glucuronide and sulfate metabolites are hepatotoxic. Rather, hepatotoxicity is believed to result from the formation of a minor but highly reactive quinone-like intermediate (1). This intermediate is normally detoxified by reaction with endogenous glutathione and eventually excreted as inactive cysteine and mercapturic acid conjugates. In instances of acetaminophen overdose, hepatic stores of glutathione become depleted and the excess reactive intermediate presumably arylates vital cell constituents, producing hepatic necrosis (1). Appropriate management of acetaminophen toxicity involves the timely oral administration of the specific therapeutic agent, N-acetylcysteine, to provide an exogenous sulfhydryl substitute for glutathione (2,3). Because the severity of acetaminophen intoxication cannot be judged clinically before the signs of toxic hepatitis appear (generally three to five days after the overdose), the decision to treat with N-acetylcysteine is based primarily on the concentration of acetaminophen in serum. Moreover, laboratory results must be available relatively quickly because the efficacy of treatment diminishes with time after the dose of acetaminophen (2,3). Nomograms have been devised relating the concentration of acetaminophen in serum according to time after ingestion and the probability of subsequent hepatic necrosis (3,4). Because these nomograms refer to the concentration of the free (unconjugated) drug, a method that measures only free acetaminophen and not the inactive glucuronide and sulfate conjugates is required (5).

The reversed-phase "high performance" liquid chromatographic (HPLC) procedure described here is rapid and simple enough for use in emergency situations and is free from common interferences.

Principle

Acetaminophen (N-acetyl-p-aminophenol) is extracted from serum with ethyl acetate and subsequently analyzed by reversed-phase HPLC with an octadecylsilane bonded-phase column. 3-Acetamidophenol (N-acetyl-m-aminophenol) is used as the internal standard and absorbance is measured at 254 nm.

Materials and Methods

Reagents

1. *Acetaminophen stock standard, 1000 mg/L.* Dissolve 100 mg of acetaminophen (USP reference standard; United States Pharmacopoeial Convention, Inc., Rockville, MD 20852, or equivalent) in 20 mL of methanol and then dilute to 100 mL with de-ionized water. Stable for at least six months when stored refrigerated.

2. *Acetaminophen working standards.* Dilute the acetaminophen stock standard with de-ionized water to provide working standards of 20 and 100 µg/mL. Stable for two months when stored refrigerated.

3. *3-Acetamidophenol stock internal standard, 1000 mg/L.* Dissolve 100 mg of 3-acetamidophenol (Aldrich Chemical Co., Inc., Milwaukee, WI 53233) in 20 mL of methanol and dilute to 100 mL with de-ionized water. Stable for six months when stored refrigerated.

4. *3-Acetamidophenol working internal standard, 50 µg/mL.* Dilute the stock internal standard 20-fold with de-ionized water. Stable for two months when stored refrigerated.

5. *Phosphate buffer, 225 mmol/L, pH 7.4.* Mix 80.4 mL of Na_2HPO_4 solution (30.6 g/L) with 19.6 mL of KH_2PO_4 solution (31.9 g/L). Adjust to pH 7.4 if necessary with the appropriate phosphate solution. Stable for two months when stored at room temperature.

6. *Sodium acetate buffer, 10 mmol/L, pH 4.0.* Dissolve 0.83 g of sodium acetate (HPLC grade; Fisher Scientific Co., Pittsburgh, PA 15219) in 1 L of de-ionized water. Adjust to pH 4.0 with glacial acetic acid. Prepare as needed for preparation of mobile phase.

7. *Mobile phase: sodium acetate buffer/acetonitrile (92/8 by vol).* Add 80 mL of acetonitrile (HPLC grade, Fisher Scientific Co.) to a 1-L volumetric flask and dilute to volume with the sodium acetate buffer. Filter through a 0.5-µm pore-size filter disc (FHUP 04700; Millipore Corp., Bedford, MA 01730) and de-gas by sparging with nitrogen for 10 min. Store tightly capped at room temperature. Stable for at least three months.

Apparatus

We used a 4.5 mm (i.d.) × 250 mm C_{18} HPLC column with 5-µm-diameter particles (IBM Instruments Inc., Danbury, CT 06810, or comparable), attached to a 0.5-µm pore-size precolumn filter (Upchurch Scientific, Inc., Oak Harbor, WA 98277). The HPLC system consisted of a

Model 6000 A pump, and a Model U6K injector (both from Waters Associates, Inc., Milford, MA 01757), but comparable systems are suitable. Either a fixed (254 nm) or variable-wavelength detector (e.g., Waters Associates Model 450) can be used and any recorder capable of receiving a 10-mV full-scale signal.

Procedure

1. In properly labeled 13 × 100 mm disposable borosilicate glass test tubes, pipet 100 μL of each standard, control, and patient's serum.

2. Add 100 μL of the working internal standard solution (50 μg/mL) and 100 μL of phosphate buffer (225 mmol/L, pH 7.4). Mix.

3. Add 2 mL of ethyl acetate. Vortex-mix for 15 s.

4. Centrifuge all tubes for 5 min at 2000 rpm in a table-top centrifuge to separate the layers.

5. Transfer the organic (top) layer to clean, labeled 12 × 75 mm borosilicate test tubes and evaporate under a stream of dry air in a 50 °C water bath.

6. Reconstitute the contents of each tube with 100 μL of the mobile phase and inject 10 to 20 μL into the chromatograph. The HPLC settings are as follows: detector sensitivity 0.1 or 0.2 A full scale (for acetaminophen concentrations of 0 to 200 or 200 to 500 μg/mL, respectively); detector wavelength 254 nm; chart speed 0.5 cm/min; pump flow rate 1.5 mL/min.

Calculations

To quantify acetaminophen, determine the respective peak-height ratios of acetaminophen to the internal standard. Calculate a response factor (f) for each standard as follows:

$$f = \frac{\text{Peak height of internal standard}}{\text{peak height of acetaminophen}} \times \text{concn, μg/mL}$$

Average the f values for the standards and use this average f value to calculate the unknowns:

$$\text{Unknown, μg/mL} = \frac{\text{Peak height of acetaminophen}}{\text{peak height of internal standard}} \times f$$

Note: Evaluators S.W.D. and D.C.H. prefer to use three standards prepared in drug-free serum and then compute results for unknowns from a plot of peak-height ratios vs concentrations for the standard concentrations.

Results

Typical chromatograms for a standard, blank, and positive serum samples are shown in Figure 1. Under the chromatographic conditions used, acetaminophen has a retention time of 5.2 min and the internal standard, 8.2 min.

Note: Evaluators S.W.D. and D.C.H. reported retention times of 5.6 and 8.4 min for acetaminophen and internal standard, respectively, using a Waters 4.5 mm (i.d.) × 250 mm C_{18} column with 5-μm-diameter particles.

The peak-height ratio response varies linearly with acetaminophen concentrations to 500 μg/mL. However, acetaminophen concentrations greater than 200 μg/mL may produce peaks that are off-scale for full-scale sensitivity settings of 0.1 A. For such samples, one may either inject a smaller sample, change the recorder sensitivity to 0.2 A until the acetaminophen peak elutes, or dilute the original sample and re-analyze. The minimum detectable concentration of acetaminophen is 1 μg/mL (at 0.1 A sensitivity setting). Within-day precision

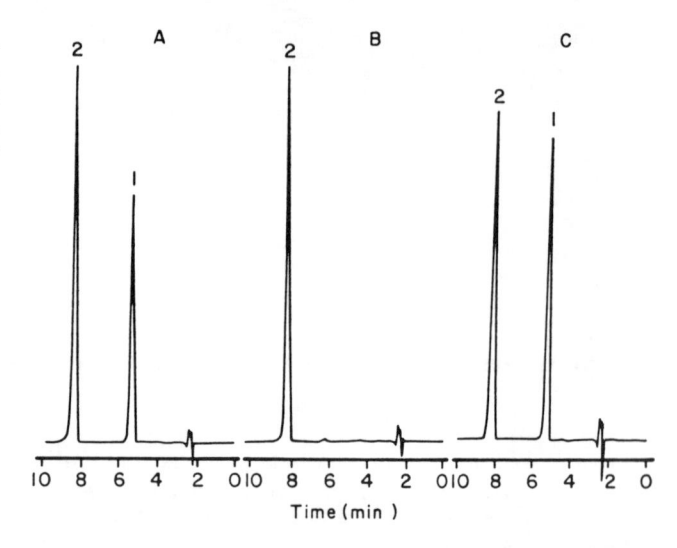

Fig. 1. Typical chromatograms for (A) acetaminophen standard (20 μg/mL), (B) acetaminophen-free serum, (C) serum containing 30 μg of acetaminophen per milliliter
1, Acetaminophen; *2*, 3-acetaminophen (internal standard)

(CV), determined with control sera containing 10 and 30 μg of acetaminophen per milliliter, was 2.5 and 2.2%, respectively. Between-day precision was 4.5% at 10 μg/mL and 4.1% at 30 μg/mL (see Table 1).

The relative analytical recovery of acetaminophen when added to bovine serum albumin (70 g/L) at concentrations of 10 and 100 μg/mL or to drug-free human serum at concentrations of 50, 100, 200, and 300 μg/mL averaged 99.6% (range, 98.3-104.1%) (Table 2). The absolute recovery was 84.6% (82.4-86.9%) at concentrations of 10 and 100 μg of acetaminophen per milliliter of bovine serum albumin solution.

We examined several drugs as possible sources of interference. When present at clinically significant concentrations, none of the drugs listed in Table 3 interfered.

Table 1. Precision Studies

	Acetaminophen, μg/mL			
	Mean	SD	CV,%	n
Within-day precision				
Evaluators S.W.D. and D.C.H.	145.7	2.8	1.9	20
Evaluator E.H.T.	9.8	0.4	4.1	4
	19.4	0.2	1.0	4
	49.1	2.3	4.7	4
Submitters	10.2	0.26	2.5	10
	30.1	0.67	2.2	10
Between-day precision				
Evaluators S.W.D. and D.C.H.	13.0	0.42	3.3	19
	140.1	5.99	4.3	20
Evaluator E.H.T.	9.8	0.5	5.1	12[a]
	19.7	1.2	6.1	12[a]
	50.9	2.1	4.1	12[a]
Submitters	10.0	0.45	4.5	20
	28.9	1.19	4.1	20

[a] Combined within-day and between-day precision (four replicates per day × three days).

Table 2. Analytical Recovery Studies

Evaluators	Acetaminophen, μg/mL	Mean recovery (and range), %
S.W.D. and D.C.H.	20, 100	98.1 (97-99.2)
Evaluator E.H.T.	10, 20, 50	99.4 (98-101.8)
Submitters	10, 50, 100, 200, 300	99.6 (98.3-104.1)

Table 3. Drugs and Compounds That Do Not Interfere with the HPLC Determination of Acetaminophen

2-Acetamidophenol	Meprobamate
Acetazolamide	Methamphetamine
N-Acetylprocainamide	Methapyrilene
Amikacin	Methaqualone
Amitryptyline	Methyprylon
Amobarbital	Nicotine
Amoxapine	Nitrazepam
Amphetamine	Norchlordiazepoxide
Atropine	Nordiazepam
Butabarbital	Norpseudoephedrine
Caffeine	Nortriptyline
Carbamazepine	Oxazepam
Chlordiazepoxide	Pentobarbital
Chlorpromazine	Phenobarbital
Codeine	Phenylpropanolamine
Demoxepam	Phenytoin
Desipramine	Procainamide
Desmethyldoxepin	Propoxyphene
Diazepam	Protriptyline
Digoxin	Pseudoephedrine
Diphenhydramine	Pyrilamine
Disopyramide	Quinidine
Doxepin	Salicylate
Ethosuximide	Secobarbital
Gentamicin	Temazepam
Glutethimide	Theobromine
β-Hydroxyethyltheophylline	Theophylline
Imipramine	Tobramycin
Lidocaine	Trimipramine
Loxapine	Valproic acid

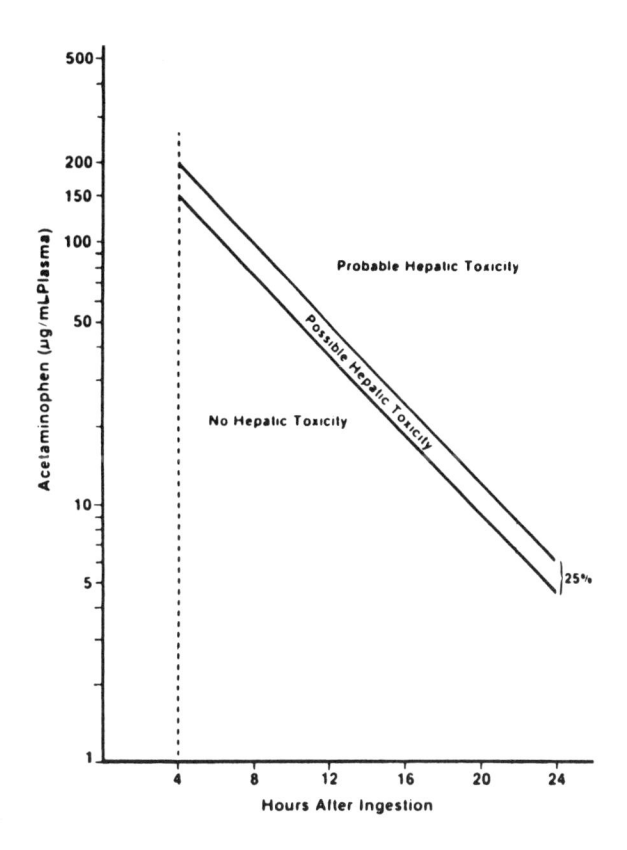

Fig. 2. Rumack-Matthew nomogram for acetaminophen poisoning

Because absorption of toxic doses may be delayed for 4 h, serum samples obtained sooner than this may not represent peak concentrations. The lower solid line 25% below the standard nomogram is included to allow for possible errors in acetaminophen assays and in estimates of the time of ingestion. From Rumack and Matthew (4), used with permission.
© American Academy of Pediatrics, 1975

Discussion

The therapeutic range for acetaminophen is 10 to 30 μg/mL (6). A high risk of serious hepatotoxicity is associated with serum concentrations of acetaminophen exceeding 200 μg/mL at 4 h post-ingestion and 50 μg/mL after 12 h (see Figure 2). An apparent drug half-life greater than 4 h has been proposed as an even better predictor of serious hepatic necrosis (7).

Acetaminophen toxicity is one of a relatively few instances of drug overdose in which there is little initial clinical indication of the severity of the intoxication but for which a specific therapeutic agent is available. Administration of N-acetylcysteine within the first 10 h after a toxic ingestion gives maximum protective efficacy (2,3), although the patient may appear quite asymptomatic during that period. However, the indiscriminate use of N-acetylcysteine is not advised (8). Therefore, the diagnosis of acetaminophen toxicity and decisions regarding therapeutic management rest on the timely laboratory determination of serum concentrations of acetaminophen by analytical methods that are both rapid and specific.

To meet this established clinical need, several different methods have been proposed for the determination of acetaminophen, including colorimetric procedures based on ring-nitration (9,10), reduction of ferric ion (11), and acid hydrolysis followed by formation of indophenol (12) or reaction with o-cresol (13). In general, these methods are relatively easy to perform but are subject to interference from acetaminophen metabolites (5, 14), salicylates and other drugs (5, 15), or endogenous substances in sera from uremic patients (16). These interferences may be significantly decreased by incorporating an extraction step before the colorimetric determination (16). The enzyme immunoassay technique (EMIT[R]; Syva Co.) and fluorescence polarization immunoassay (Abbott Laboratories) are specific and relatively easy to perform but require the use of rather expensive reagents (17,18). A new colorimetric method based on the enzymic hydrolysis of acetaminophen appears to be free from interferences (19) but also requires somewhat expensive reagents (Diagnostic Chemicals Ltd., Monroe, CT). Gas-chromatographic procedures are sensitive and specific but generally require silylation or alkylation to avoid adsorption onto the column and tailing of peaks *(20,21)*. Methods based on HPLC do not require derivatization and are relatively simple and specific *(22-25)*. The HPLC method described here offers advantages of simplicity, selection of internal standard, and freedom from interferences. We therefore recommend it for those laboratories that have the required instrumentation.

Note: Evaluators S.W.D. and D.C.H. obtained comparable results with the HPLC method and the enzyme immunoassay technique (EMIT) for a limited number of patients' specimens. Evaluator E.H.T. obtained similar results with the HPLC method and the colorimetric method of Glynn and Kendal *(9)* for serum samples to which acetaminophen had been added.

References

1. Mitchell JR, Thorgeirsson SS, Potter WZ, et al. Acetaminophen-induced hepatic injury: Protective role of glutathione in man and rationale for therapy. *Clin Pharmacol Ther* **16**, 676-684 (1974).
2. Rumack BH, Peterson RG. Acetaminophen overdose: Incidence, diagnosis, and management in 416 patients. *Pediatrics* **62**, 898-903 (1978).
3. Rumack BH, Peterson RC, Kock GG, Amara IA. Acetaminophen overdose: 662 cases with evaluation of oral acetylcysteine treatment. *Arch Intern Med* **141**, 380-385 (1981).
4. Rumack BH, Matthew H. Acetaminophen poisoning and toxicity. *Pediatrics* **55**, 871-876 (1975).
5. Stewart MJ, Adriaenssenes P, Jarvie D, Prescott L. Inappropriate methods for the emergency determination of plasma paracetamol. *Ann Clin Biochem* **16**, 89-95 (1979).
6. Tietz NW (Ed). *Clinical Guide to Laboratory Tests*, WB Saunders Co., Philadelphia, PA, 1983, p 562.
7. Prescott LF, Roscoe P, Wright N, Brown SS. Plasma paracetamol half-life and hepatic necrosis in patients with paracetamol overdosage. *Lancet* **i**, 519-522 (1971).
8. Ambre J, Alexander M. Liver toxicity after acetaminophen ingestion: Inadequacy of the dose estimate as an index of risk. *J Am Med Assoc* **238**, 500-501 (1977).
9. Glynn JP, Kendal SE. Paracetamol measurement. *Lancet* **i**, 1147-1148 (1975).
10. Walberg CB. Determination of acetaminophen in serum. *J Anal Tox* **1**, 79-80 (1977).
11. Liu TZ, Oka KH. Spectrometric screening method for acetaminophen in serum and plasma. *Clin Chem* **26**, 69-71 (1980).
12. Frings CS, Saloom JM. Colorimetric method for the quantitative determination of acetaminophen in serum. *Clin Toxicol* **15**, 67-73 (1979).
13. Miceli JN, Aravind MK. A rapid, simple acetaminophen determination is available. *Clin Chem* **26**, 1627 (1980). Letter.
14. Buttery JE, Braiotta EA, Pannall PR. Plasma acetaminophen results are method dependent. *J Toxicol Clin Toxicol* **19**, 1117-1122 (1982-83).
15. Buttery JE, Braiotta EA, Pannall PR. Correction for salicylate interference in the colorimetric paracetamol assay. *Clin Chim Acta* **122**, 301-304 (1983).
16. Bailey DN. Colorimetry of serum acetaminophen (paracetamol) in uremia. *Clin Chem* **28**, 187-190 (1982).
17. Bridges RR, Kinniburgh DW, Keehn BJ, Jennison TA. An evaluation of common methods for acetaminophen quantitation for small hospitals. *Clin Toxicol* **20**, 1-17 (1983).
18. Keegan C, Smith C, Ungemach F, Simpson J. A fluorescence polarization immunoassay for the quantitation of acetaminophen. *Clin Chem* **30**, 1025 (1984). Abstract.
19. Price CP, Hammond PM, Scawen MD. Evaluation of an enzymic procedure for the measurement of acetaminophen. *Clin Chem* **29**, 358-361 (1983).
20. Prescott LF. The gas-liquid chromatographic estimation of phenacetin and paracetamol in plasma and urine. *J Pharm Pharmacol* **23**, 111-115 (1971).
21. Dechtiaruk WA, Johnson GF, Solomon HM. Gas chromatographic method for acetaminophen (*N*-acetyl-*p*-aminophenol) based on sequential alkylation. *Clin Chem* **22**, 879-883 (1976).
22. Gotelli GR, Kabra PM, Marton LJ. Determination of acetaminophen and phenacetin in plasma by high-pressure liquid chromatography. *Clin Chem* **23**, 957-959 (1977).
23. Horvitz RA, Jatlow PI. Determination of acetaminophen concentrations in serum by high pressure liquid chromatography. *Clin Chem* **23**, 1596-1598 (1977).
24. Fletterick CG, Grove TH, Hohnadel DC. Liquid-chromatographic determination of acetaminophen in serum. *Clin Chem* **25**, 409-412 (1979).
25. Miceli JN, Aravind MK, Cohen SN, Done AK. Simultaneous measurements of acetaminophen and salicylate in plasma by liquid chromatography. *Clin Chem* **25**, 1002-1004 (1979).

Acetaminophen by Colorimetry

Submitters: Frank M. Stearns and Robert W. Dalrymple, *Damon Clinical Laboratories, Trevose, PA 19047*

Evaluator: Larry A. Broussard, *Medical Laboratory Associates, Birmingham, AL 35256*

Introduction

Acetaminophen (*N*-acetyl-*p*-aminophenol) was introduced as an antipyretic analgesic in Europe in 1893 under the name paracetamol. It was not widely used until after 1949, when it was shown that the major metabolites of two generally used analgesics, phenacetin and acetanilide, are rapidly metabolized to acetaminophen. Since then this drug has gained wide acceptance and since 1955 has been available in the United States without a prescription. Acetaminophen has been marketed under more than 50 brand names, such as Tylenol, Tempra, Datril, and Liquiprin, and in almost 200 more proprietary combinations with other compounds, e.g., Darvocet-N, Excedrin, Sinutab, and Bromo Seltzer.

Acetaminophen has successfully replaced aspirin as an analgesic/antipyretic because it lacks many of aspirin's side effects. Because of its general availability in the home, acute acetaminophen overdoses are common in adults attempting suicide. As with aspirin, massive overdose with acetaminophen can be toxic and potentially fatal.

Ingestion of a single 10- to 15-g dose of acetaminophen has produced hepatotoxicity in adults, and a dose of 25 g or more is potentially fatal. Symptoms during the first 48 h of acute poisoning do not reflect the potential severity of the toxicity.

The need to monitor the concentrations of acetaminophen in serum has been well documented (1-3), and spectrophotometric (4-8), gas-liquid chromatographic (9-11), liquid chromatographic (12-14), enzymic colorimetric (15), and enzymic immunoassay (EMIT) (16) methods have been developed for its determination. Colorimetric methods involving nitration of *N*-acetyl-*p*-aminophenol are widely used because of the simplicity, rapidity, and range of linearity of this reaction. Interference by salicylate is a problem but can be compensated for by using a correction factor.

The method described here was originally reported by Frings and Saloom (17) and has been used in the Submitters' laboratory for five years. The method is simple and rapid, is not subject to interference from salicylate, and can be used to quantify acetaminophen in therapeutic as well as toxic situations.

Note: The Editors are aware of the controversy (18,19) regarding this type of method. The method presented here does not give false-negative results, but can overestimate acetaminophen in serum, especially in patients with renal disease. High values for acetaminophen should be interpreted with caution in patients with high concentrations of urea and (or) creatinine. This method has been useful in laboratories without facilities for "high-performance" liquid chromatography.

Principle

A protein-free filtrate is prepared from serum by adding trichloroacetic acid. An aliquot of the filtrate is then boiled with hydrochloric acid to hydrolyze the *N*-acetyl-*p*-aminophenol (acetaminophen) to *p*-aminophenol. The *p*-aminophenol reacts with phenol and ammonium hydroxide to form an indophenol blue chromogen. The absorbance of this chromogen at 620 nm follows Beer's law for acetaminophen concentrations up to 50 mg/L.

Materials and Methods

Reagents

1. *Trichloroacetic acid,* 200 g/L: Dissolve 200 g of trichloroacetic acid in water and dilute to 1 L. The solution is stable for six months stored in a brown glass bottle at 4-7 °C.

2. *Concentrated hydrochloric acid:* Reagent grade.

3. *Ammonium hydroxide,* 4 mol/L: Dilute 142 mL of concentrated ammonium hydroxide to volume with water in a 500-mL volumetric flask. The solution is stable for two months stored in a brown glass bottle at room temperature.

4. *Phenol,* 20 g/L: Mix 23 mL of liquified phenol in water and dilute to 1000 mL with water in a volumetric flask. The solution is stable for four months stored in a brown glass bottle at 4-7 °C. Do not use phenol crystals to prepare this reagent.

5. *Color reagent:* Mix seven volumes of the phenol reagent with three volumes of the ammonium hydroxide reagent. Prepare a fresh solution just before use.

6. *Acetaminophen stock standard,* 1000 mg/L: Dissolve 100 mg of acetaminophen (McNeil Laboratories, Inc., Fort Washington, PA 19034) in water and dilute to 100 mL with water in a volumetric flask. This standard is stable stored for six months in a brown glass bottle at 4-7 °C.

7. *Acetaminophen working standards,* 0, 12.5, 25, and 50 mg/L: Using pooled blank serum and 100-mL volumetric flasks, dilute to volume the appropriate

amount of acetaminophen stock solution (see below). Freeze these working standards in 3.0-mL aliquots; they are stable for one year.

Vol, mL		Final concn of acetaminophen standard, mg/L
Stock acetaminophen	Pooled serum	
0.0	100	0.0
1.25	98.75	12.5
2.5	97.5	25.0
5.0	95.0	50.0

Collection and Handling of Specimens

Serum samples are required for the analysis for acetaminophen. Specimens need not be refrigerated and are stable for approximately seven days. Specimens should be obtained upon admission to the hospital, especially if the drug was ingested within the previous 4 h. A second specimen should be taken 4 h later. The half-life should be determined from the 4-h and 8-h determinations.

Procedure

1. Pipet 1.0 mL of blank (zero standard), standards, controls, and unknowns into labeled 16 × 100 mm glass test tubes.
2. Add 2.0 mL of trichloroacetic acid reagent to each tube, vortex-mix for 5 s, and centrifuge until a clear supernate is obtained.
3. Transfer 1.0 mL of the clear supernate from each tube to properly labeled 16 × 100 mm glass test tubes.
4. Add 0.2 mL of concentrated hydrochloric acid to each tube and place in a boiling water bath for at least 20 min but not more than 30 min.
5. Remove the tubes from the water bath, then add 5.0 mL of freshly prepared color reagent to each tube and vortex-mix for 5 s.
6. After 30 min, but before 1 h, read the absorbance of the standards and unknowns at 620 nm in a 1-cm cuvet vs the blank.

Results and Discussion

Linearity and sensitivity. A plot of four concentrations of aqueous standards taken through the entire procedure formed a straight line to at least 50 mg of acetaminophen per liter. The correlation coefficient was 0.998. Least-squares linear regression analysis yielded a slope of 0.041. As little as 1 mg of acetaminophen per liter can be reproducibly quantified.

> *Note:* Evaluator L.A.B. reports that a linear curve is obtained when absorbance is plotted vs serum acetaminophen concentrations up to 500 mg/L in samples taken through the entire procedure.

Analytical recovery. The recovery of acetaminophen from serum was approximately 80% when compared with aqueous standards. The recovery is increased to 100% when serum-based standards are used (17).

Precision. Intra-assay precision was evaluated by processing aliquots of frozen pooled serum containing acetaminophen at two concentrations. The CV was 6.8% (n = 10) for acetaminophen at a mean concentration of 14.9 mg/L and 3.8% (n = 10) at a mean concentration of 46.9 mg/L. Interassay CV (n = 21) at mean acetaminophen concentrations of 15.2 and 45.8 mg/L was 9.5% and 6.5%, respectively.

Interference. Potential interferences from other drugs were investigated by taking through the entire procedure a solution of each drug listed in Table 1. All of the drugs were tested at a concentration of 100 mg/L except sodium bromide (1000 mg/L), caffeine (1000 mg/L), chloral hydrate (500 mg/L), and chlorpheniramine (80 mg/L). None interfered with the method.

Table 1. Drugs That Do Not Interfere with Determinations of Acetaminophen

Acetazolamide	Mephenesin carbamate
Amitriptyline	Mephobarbital
Amobarbital	Meprobamate
Amoxapine	Methadone
Amphetamine	Methamphetamine
Barbital	Methaqualone
Bromide, Na	Methsuximide
Butabarbital	Methylphenidate
Caffeine	Methyprylon
Carbamazepine	Morphine
Carisoprodol	Oxazepam
Chloral hydrate	Pemoline
Chlordiazepoxide	Pentazocine
Chlorpheniramine	Pentobarbital
Chlorpromazine	Perphenazine
Clorazepate	Phenacetin
Cocaine	Phencyclidine
Codeine	Phenmetrazine
Diazepam	Phenobarbital
Diflunisal	Phenylephrine
Diphenhydramine	Phenylpropanolamine
Disulfiram	Phenytoin
Doxepin	Primadone
Ephedrine	Primaquine
Ethanol	Procainamide
Ethchlorvynol	Propoxyphene
Ethosuximide	Propranolol
Fenfluramine	Pyrilamine
Fluphenazine	Quinidine
Flurazepam	Salicylate, Na
Gentamicin	Secobarbital
Glutethimide	Sulfanilamide
Haloperidol	Theophylline
Hydromorphone	Thiopropazate
Imipramine	Thioridazine
Isoniazid	Thiothixene
Loxapine	Trazodone
Mebutamate	Trifluoperazine
Meperidine	Triflupromazine
Mephenesin	

See text for concentrations tested.

Therapeutic range. After therapeutic administration of 8-10 mg/kg for children, and 10-20 mg/kg for adults, the concentrations of acetaminophen in serum are usually 10-20 and 10-30 mg/L, respectively.

Minimal hepatotoxicity is produced when the serum concentration is less than 120 mg/L at 4 h after ingestion, or less than 50 mg/L after 12 h. The half-life (t½) may be used to judge toxicity, the usual t½ being 2 to 3 h. When the t½ exceeds 4 h, liver damage is probable and treatment with N-acetylcysteine (antidote) is indicated. A useful nomograph for the assessment of potential acetaminophen toxicity has been published (20).

Shortly after this manuscript was completed, Novotny and Elser (21) reported a modification of the procedure just described. They suggested that, because of insufficient acid concentration and hydrolysis time, the rate of conversion of acetominophen to p-aminophenol was less than complete; they therefore recommended additional acidification of the trichloroacetic acid supernate with hydrochloric acid, and increasing the incubation time to 35 min.

Although the modified procedure indicates a need for a greater acid concentration, review of both procedures with respect to final HCl concentration showed no difference, the effective HCl concentration being 2.0 mol/L in each.

Novotny and Elser also recommended increasing the heating step to 35 min to ensure complete hydrolysis, although they demonstrated that hydrolysis is essentially complete at 20 min. Their report is consistent with our recommendation for a hydrolysis time of 20-30 min.

References

1. Peterson RG, Rumack BH. Treating acute acetaminophen poisoning with acetylcysteine. *J Am Med Assoc* **237**, 2406-2407 (1977).
2. Krenzelok EP, Best L, Manoguerra AS. Acetaminophen toxicity. *Am J Hosp Pharm* **34**, 391-394 (1977).
3. Smith FA. Therapeutic drug monitoring of theophylline, salicylates, and acetaminophen. *Clin Lab Med* **1**, 559-579 (1980).
4. Chafetz L, Daly RE, Schriftman H, Lomner JJ. Selective colorimetric determination of acetaminophen. *J Pharm Sci* **60**, 463-466 (1971).
5. Kendal SE, Lloyd-Jones G, Smith CF. The development of a blood paracetamol estimation kit. *J Int Med Res* **4**, 83-88 (1976).
6. Walberg CB. Determination of acetaminophen in serum. *J Anal Toxicol* **1**, 79-80 (1977).
7. Routh JI, Shane NA, Arrendo EG, Paul WD. Determination of N-acetyl-p-aminophenol in plasma. *Clin Chem* **14**, 882-889 (1968).
8. Knefil J. A sensitive specific method for measuring N-acetyl-p-aminophenol (paracetamol) in blood. *Clin Chim Acta* **52**, 369-372 (1974).
9. Grove J. Gas liquid chromatography of N-acetyl-p-aminophenol (paracetamol) in plasma and urine. *J Chromatogr* **59**, 289-295 (1971).
10. Prescott LF. The gas-liquid chromatographic estimation of phenacetin in plasma and urine. *J Pharm Pharmacol* **23**, 111-115 (1971).
11. Dechtiaruk WA, Johnson GF, Solomon HM. Gas chromatographic method for acetaminophen (N-acetyl-p-aminophenol) based on sequential alkylation. *Clin Chem* **22**, 879-883 (1976).
12. Black M, Sprague K. Rapid micromethod for acetaminophen determination. *Clin Chem* **24**, 1288-1289 (1978).
13. Blair D, Rumack BH. Acetaminophen in serum and plasma estimated by high-pressure liquid chromatography: A micro-scale method. *Clin Chem* **23**, 743-745 (1977).
14. Fletterick CG, Grove TH, Hohnadel DC. Liquid chromatographic determination of acetaminophen in serum. *Clin Chem* **25**, 409-412 (1979).
15. Price CP, Hammond PM, Schawen MD. Evaluation of an enzymic procedure for the measurement of acetaminophen. *Clin Chem* **29**, 358-361 (1983).
16. Masover B, DeLaurentis M, Turner J. EMIT® - tox acetaminophen assay, clinical study no. 106, summary report. Syva Co., Palo Alto, CA, 1982.
17. Frings CS, Saloom M. Colorimetric method for the quantitative determination of acetaminophen in serum. *Clin Toxicol* **15**, 67-73 (1979).
18. Stewart MJ, Adriaenssens P, Jarvie D, Prescott L. Inappropriate methods for the emergency determination of plasma paracetamol. *Ann Clin Biochem* **16**, 89-95 (1979).
19. Porter WH. In acetaminophen assays, only unconjugated drug should be measured. *Clin Chem* **30**, 1884-1885 (1984). Letter.
20. Rumack BH, Matthew H. Acetaminophen poisoning and toxicity. *Pediatrics* **55**, 871-876 (1975).
21. Novotny PE, Elser RC. Indophenol method for acetaminophen in serum examined. *Clin Chem* **30**, 884-886 (1984).

Alcohols in Biological Fluids by Gas Chromatography (Automated Head-Space Method)

Submitters: Richard H. Gadsden, Sr., and C. Steven Terry, *Department of Laboratory Medicine, Medical University of South Carolina, Charleston, SC 29425*

Evaluator: Bernard C. Thompson, *Department of Toxicology, SmithKline Bioscience Laboratories, Inc., King of Prussia, PA 19406*

Introduction

The clinical laboratory is frequently responsible for analysis of biological fluids for the detection and quantification of alcohol. Clinically, this is important in monitoring patients under an alcohol-restrictive protocol, in drug-abuse programs, and for emergency care. With the traumatized patient, where use of anesthetics before surgery is anticipated, the attending physician must know whether the patient has imbibed alcohol and, if so, what type(s) and quantities are present. Often speed is required.

Enzymic analysis for alcohol in biological fluid has been well worked out (1), but these methods are relatively highly specific for ethanol. Freezing-point osmometry coupled with enzymic alcohol analysis (2) corroborates the presence of a volatile intoxicant and can rapidly determine intrinsic causes of metabolic intoxification. However, although this method is rapid to perform, it does not specifically identify the volatile intoxicant present other than ethanol. Gas chromatography, on the other hand, is ideally suited for differentiating and quantifying volatile substances (low-M_r alcohols and acetone) in a sample (3).

The best gas-chromatographic analysis for alcohols involves head-space analysis (4,5), a method amenable to and enhanced by computerized automation (6). This approach greatly prolongs the life of the column and obviates contamination of the detector. We have found this method useful for the determination of volatile substances in solid samples (e.g., organs, such as liver and brain) as well as biological fluids.

Principle

Volatile compounds of relatively high vapor pressure that are frequently encountered in clinical medicine are methanol, ethanol, acetone, and isopropanol. Gas-chromatographic head-space analysis is eminently suitable for analysis of these compounds in biological samples containing a large proportion of nonvolatile materials. With proper standardization the technique permits identification of the volatile component(s) and quantification. Computerized automation enhances throughput and analytical precision.

The sample to be analyzed is quantitatively transferred to a vial, an aliquot of internal standard is added, and the vial is tightly sealed. The vial is placed in a thermostated sample block, and sample and the vapor in the vial head-space are allowed to reach equilibrium. The sample vial is then pressurized with carrier gas, after which an aliquot of the vapor contents is injected onto the gas-chromatographic column. The entire analytical procedure—thermostatic equilibrium, sample injection, chromatography, and identification/calculation—is sequenced by the computer.

Materials and Methods

Apparatus

We use a Model F-45 head-space analyzer (Perkin-Elmer Corp., Instrument Division, Norwalk, CT 06856). This equipment is modular and consists of the following components: chromatographic column, oven, thermostated turntable for the samples, and head-space sample injector; temperature-control module for setting temperatures (°C) of the oven, injector, and flame-ionization detector (FID); head-space programmer for sample sequencing, sample pressurization and injection time, analysis time, column back-flush time (necessary if the volatilized sample contains high-boiling components), injector needle dwell time, and stabilization time; head-space power supply; an FID amplifier; an FID gas module (for regulation of the air and hydrogen supply to the FID); a Model M-1 computing integrator for automatic identification and calculation of concentration of alcohols, based on previous standardization; and (optional) a recorder (Fisher Scientific, Pittsburgh, PA 15219; Fisher Recordall, cat. no. 14-939-10) for graphic display of the chromatographic separation of the volatilized sample components.

The sample vial unit (Perkin-Elmer) consists of a vial (cat. no. 0105-0129), star washer, rubber septum, and cap (cat. no. 0105-0131).

Chromatographic Conditions

Column: 6 ft. × 1/8 in. (183 cm × 3 mm, i.d.) stainless steel packed with 0.2% Carbowax 1500 on 60/80-mesh Carbopak C (available from Perkin-Elmer). Temperatures: sample turntable, 70 °C; injector and needle, 150 °C; chromotograph oven, 150 °C. Carrier gas, nitrogen; flow rate, 35 mL/min. FID gases: air, 3.6 mL/min; hydrogen, 2.8 mL/min. FID programmer: range, 10; attenuation, 4. Head-space programmer times: sample, 2 s; chromatography, 4 min; column flush, 15 s. Computing integrator: program 2. Recorder chart speed: 1 cm/min.

Standards

Ethanol stock standard. All pipetting and weighing are performed at room temperature. Pre-weigh a 50-mL GS volumetric flask containing about 25 mL of distilled (or de-ionized) water (this avoids the absorption of atmospheric water when absolute ehtanol is added to the flask). Add 5 mL of absolute ethanol (reagent quality; AAPER Alcohol & Chemical Co., Shelbyville, KY 40065), and reweigh. Determine the weight of the ethanol by the difference. Dilute to 50 mL with distilled water. This stock standard is stable indefinitely when refrigerated and protected against evaporation. Before preparing working standards, bring a suitable volume of stock standard to room temperature.

Ethanol working standards. Pipet 5, 4, 3, 2, and 1 mL of the ethanol stock standard into individual 100-mL GS volumetric flasks and add distilled water to volume. Mix well by inversion. Protected against evaporation and refrigerated, these standards are stable indefinitely.

Example: At room temperature (20 °C), 4 mL of the weighed ethanol ($d = 0.78945$) should weigh 3.1578 g (7). The concentrations of the working standards should thus be 3947, 3158, 2368, 1579, and 790 mg/L, respectively.

Internal standard. Dilute 1.6 mL of n-propanol (reagent grade) to 100 mL with distilled water. Stable when refrigerated.

Composite control. This is used primarily to assure proper chromatographic sequencing of the volatile analyte constituents (Figure 1).

Ethanol stock control: Pipet 2.6 mL of reagent-grade ethanol into a 100-mL GS volumetric flask and dilute to volume with distilled water: final concentration is about 2053 mg/L. Stable (refrigerated).

Methanol stock control: Pipet 2.6 mL of reagent-grade methanol into a 100-mL GS volumetric flask and dilute to volume with distilled water. Final concentration is approximately 2058 mg/L. Stable (refrigerated).

Isopropanol stock control: Pipet 2.6 mL of reagent-grade isopropanol into a 100-mL GS volumetric flask and dilute to volume with distilled water. Final concentration is approximately 2042 mg/L. Stable (refrigerated).

Acetone stock control: Pipet 2.6 mL of reagent-grade acetone into a 100-mL GS volumetric flask and dilute to volume with distilled water. Final concentration is approximately 2054 mg/L. Stable (regrigerated).

Working composite control. Pipet 10 mL each of the stock control solutions of ethanol, methanol, and isopropanol and 2.5 mL of the acetone stock control solutions into a 100-mL GS volumetric flask and dilute to volume with distilled water. Final concentrations are about 2000 mg/L for each alcohol and 500 mg/L for acetone.

Note: Stock control solutions for methanol, isopropanol, and acetone, if prepared accurately by weight/volume, can be serially diluted and used as standards, like the ethanol standards.

Method

Standardize the chromatograph according to the manufacturer's direction (8), using the ethanol working standard, internal standard, and working control materials described above. Then use the following method for calibration and for determining unknowns.

Before running an analysis of a single unknown, analyze the working composite control and the 1579 mg/L ethanol working standard. When analyzing multiple unknowns, we recommend including the ethanol working standard after about every eight unknowns and concluding the run with the working composite control.

Prepare vials as follows: for the control vial, mix 1 mL of the working composite control and 100 µL of the internal standard; for the standard vial, mix 1 mL of the ethanol working standard and 100 µL of the internal standard; for the unknowns, mix 1 mL of unknown (blood, serum/plasma, cerebrospinal fluid, or vitreous fluid) and 100 µL of the internal standard. Cover each vial, in order, with a septum, a star washer, and a cap. Crimp the cap tightly onto the vial.

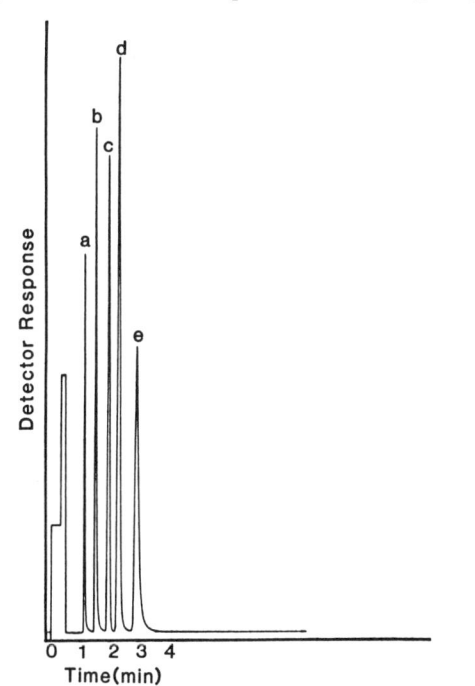

Fig. 1. The gas-chromatographic sequencing of the working composite standard: (*a*) methanol; (*b*) ethanol; (*c*) acetone; (*d*) isopropanol; (*e*) n-propanol, the internal standard

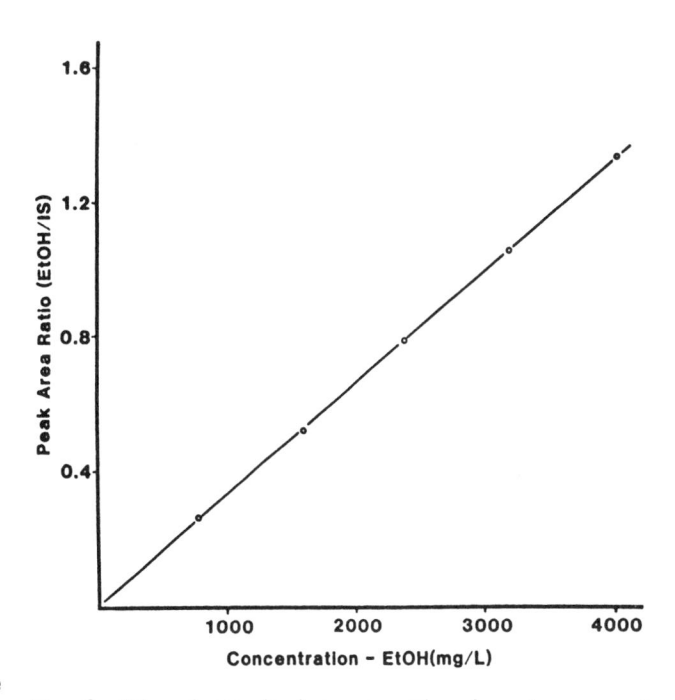

Fig. 2. Ethanol standard curve: ratio of peak areas of ethanol standards to the peak area of the internal standard plotted vs ethanol concentration

Table 1. Gas-Chromatographic Retention Times (seconds)

Analyte	Submitters' data						Evaluator's data					
	Within-run (n = 12)			Run-to-run (n = 22)			Within-run (n = 20)			Run-to-run (n = 20)		
	Mean	SD	CV, %	Mean	SD	CV, %	Mean	SD	CV, %	Mean	SD	CV, %
Methanol	37.73	0.452	1.20	37.75	0.456	1.21	39	0.0	0.0	39	0.0	0.0
Ethanol	60.27	0.456	0.76	60.33	0.492	0.82	57	0.0	0.0	57	0.03	0.52
Acetone	86.67	0.477	0.55	86.68	0.493	0.57	83	0.004	0.48	83	0.0	0.0
Isopropanol	107.23	0.491	0.46	107.33	0.527	0.49	95	0.0	0.0	95	0.0	0.0
Internal std. (n-propanol)	143.75	0.500	0.35	143.82	0.622	0.43	121	0.0	0.0	121	0.04	0.33

Place the vials on the thermostated sample turntable and let them come to equilibrium for 30 min, then initiate the automated analysis. Identify peaks by comparing the retention times with those of the standards.

Calculation

The calculation is based on the ratio of the peak area of the analyte to that for the internal standard. This varies linearly with concentration (Figure 2). If an integrator is not available, calculate the analyte concentration on the basis of the ratio of the peak height (PH) for the analyte to that for the internal standard (IS).

Example: Calculate the concentration of ethanol in a sample as follows:

$$\text{Concn in sample} = \frac{\text{PH of ethanol, sample}}{\text{PH of IS, sample}} \times \frac{\text{PH of IS, std.}}{\text{PH of ethanol, std.}} \times \text{concn of ethanol in std.}$$

Results

Precision

Table 1 illustrates the within-run and run-to-run precision with respect to the retention times for methanol, ethanol, isopropanol, and acetone in the working composite control, as determined with the automated head-space gas-chromatographic system.

Table 2 summarizes the precision of within-run analyses by peak-area ratios for 12 individually prepared samples of the working composite control run sequentially. These data also indicate the precision for run-to-run analyses by peak-area ratios for 22 individually prepared samples of the working composite control that were incorporated into routine analytical runs for blood alcohol over a one-month period. Also shown are the Evaluators' precision data for peak-area ratios for a composite control in whole blood.

Recovery

Table 3 indicates the analytical recovery of the alcohols and acetone from prepared whole-blood samples. Solutions containing known amounts of ethanol were prepared by pipeting 5, 4, 3, 2, and 1 mL of the ethanol stock standard into individual 10-mL GS volumetric flasks and diluting to volume with distilled water. We used a pooled whole-blood sample with EDTA as anticoagulant and with no alcohols or detectable acetone to prepare standards as follows: We mixed 0.9 mL of blood with 0.1 mL of each ethanol concentration and 100 µL of internal standard solution. The sample vials were sealed and chromatographed as described above. We made 10 sequential runs in duplicate of each prepared sample. Similarly, we prepared and assayed whole-blood samples containing methanol acetone, and isopropanol at the concentrations noted in Table 3.

Table 2. Within-Run and Run-to-Run Precision for Analysis of the Composite Working Control

Analyte	Peak-area ratio			Concn, mg/L		
	Mean	SD	CV, %	Mean	SD	CV, %
Submitters' data							
Within-run (n = 12)						
Methanol	0.345	0.003	1.01	2168	29.1	1.32
Ethanol	0.725	0.008	1.03	2136	23.7	1.12
Isopropanol	1.403	0.017	1.23	2044	30.5	1.51
Acetone	0.855	0.017	2.04	517	13.3	2.23
Run-to-run (n = 22)						
Methanol	0.349	0.008	2.43	2155	54.5	2.53
Ethanol	0.722	0.010	1.32	2140	33.5	1.57
Isopropanol	1.391	0.038	2.75	2049	48.4	2.36
Acetone	0.865	0.024	2.72	510	14.6	2.48
Evaluator's data[a]						
Within-run (n = 20)						
Methanol	0.177	0.02	1.13	780	11	1.41
Ethanol	0.652	0.07	1.07	1430	16	1.11
Isopropanol	0.681	0.07	1.03	770	8	1.03
Acetone	0.659	0.14	2.12	315	7	2.22
Run-to-run (n = 20)						
Methanol	0.183	0.05	2.73	780	14	1.79
Ethanol	0.668	0.14	2.10	1430	22	1.53
Isopropanol	0.693	0.17	2.45	760	11	1.44
Acetone	0.636	0.25	3.93	337	27	8.01

[a] Whole-blood composite control.

Figure 3 illustrates interlaboratory reproducibility of the method. Twenty plasma samples and 20 whole-blood samples analyzed in the Submitters' laboratory were fowarded to the Evaluator's laboratory without indication of the results. Both sets of results were analyzed statistically and compared.

In the Submitters' laboratory the mean ($\pm$SD) results for ethanol were 178.9 (74.2) mg/dL in whole blood, 194.0 (78.4) mg/dL in plasma. Evaluator B.C.T. obtained respective results of 176.5 (73.2) and 192.5 (78.0) mg/dL. The correlation between the Evaluator's results (y) and the Submitters' data (x) was for whole blood, $y = 0.986 x + 0.629$ mg/dL ($r = 0.997$), and for plasma, $y = 0.993 x - 0.187$ mg/dL ($r = 0.999$).

Discussion

Head-space gas chromatography is ideal for qualitative and quantitative analysis of the low-boiling-point aliphatic alcohols and acetone in biological fluids. The method is accurate and precise, and can be used for analysis of alcohols in solid tissue.

Table 3. Analytical Recovery of Alcohols and Acetone from Whole Blood

Ethanol, mg/L				Methanol, mg/L			
Expected	Measured mean (SD)	Range	CV, %	Expected	Measured mean (SD)	Range	CV, %
3947	3937 (52)	3850-4036	1.32	2000	2016 (6)	2010-2024	0.30
3158	3150 (62)	3071-3245	1.96	1500	1495 (14)	1480-1509	0.93
2368	2368 (15)	2342-2392	0.65	1000	1012 (13)	996-1022	1.33
1579	1578 (17)	1554-1604	1.10	400	408 (6)	398-415	1.57
790	789 (13)	769-811	1.65				

Acetone, mg/L				Ispropanol, mg/L			
Expected	Measured mean (SD)	Range	CV, %	Expected	Measured mean (SD)	Range	CV, %
1400	1405 (19)	1377-1424	1.39	1976	1980 (3)	1950-2028	1.56
560	563 (5)	558-570	0.93	1482	1483 (4)	1478-1486	0.23
350	354 (7)	346-363	2.03	988	988 (4)	983-993	0.42
175	176 (1)	176-179	0.73	395	393 (3)	389-396	0.71

n = 20 each.

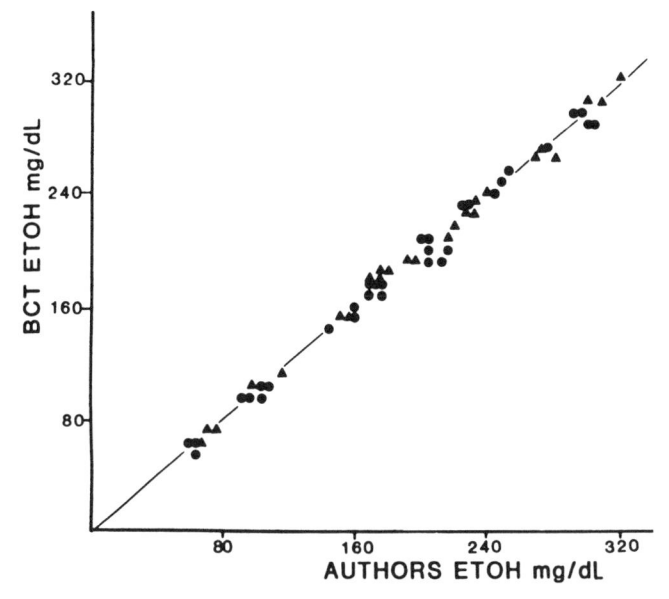

Fig. 3. Correlation of interlaboratory analysis of plasma (▲) and whole-blood (●) ethanol by gas-chromatographic head-space analysis
The line shown is y = x. BCT, Evaluator B.C.T.

Using head-space methodology prolongs the life of the chromatographic column. The Submitters have made more than 10 000 on-column injections of vapor samples and have not experienced loss of column resolution.

The chromatography is simple and takes little time, making the method amenable to rapid sample assessment and application to patient care.

References

1. Redetzki HM, Dees WL. Comparison of four kits for enzymatic determination of ethanol in blood. *Clin Chem* **22**, 83-86 (1976).
2. Pappas AA, Gadsden RH Jr, Gadsden RH Sr, Groves WE. Computerized calculation of osmolality and its automatic comparison to observed ethanol concentration. *Am J Clin Pathol* **77**, 449-451 (1982).
3. Dubowski K. Ethanol-type C procedure. In *Methodology for Analytical Toxicology*, I Sunshine, Ed., CRC Press Inc., Boca Raton, FL 33409, 1971, pp 149-154.
4. Macheta G. Advantages of automated alcohol determination by headspace analysis. *Reichmed* **75**, 229-234 (1975).
5. Machata G. Uber die gas-gaschromatographische Blutalkohol-Bestimmung. *Blutalkohol* **4**, 3-11 (1967).
6. Battista HJ. Computerized blood alcohol analysis. *Chromatographia* **5**, 206-208 (1972)
7. *Handbook of Chemistry and Physics,* 62nd ed. (1981-82), CRC Press, Boca Raton, FL 33409, p F-3 (table).
8. *Instructions: Model 1 Computing Integrator* (1975 revision), Perkin-Elmer Corp., Norwalk, CT 06856. Section 6: Internal standard. Method 2C, pp 6-9 to 6-10 and 6-36 to 6-39.

Arsenic by Spectrophotometry (Provisional)[1]

Submitter: C. Ray Ratliff, *Bio-Analytic Laboratories, Inc., Palm City, FL 33490*

Introduction

Arsenic, second only to lead as a chronic poison, is reportedly the heavy metal most frequently found reponsible for acute poisoning (*1*). Most acute and chronic arsenic poisoning cases seen today result from accidental ingestion of arsenicals in insecticides and herbicides or from industrial exposure. Phosphate detergents have also been accused of introducing arsenic into the water supply (*2,3*).

In the past, arsenic was usually determined in clinical or postmortem material by the Gutzeit or Reinsch screening procedures. Although sensitive, the Gutzeit method does not always produce distinctly colored reactions for quantification. In 1961, an easier colorimetric procedure (*4*) was reported, but it required pretreatment of urine specimens before analysis. This colorimetric procedure was then modified to measure urinary arsenic directly without wet ashing (*5*). Except for neutron activation analysis, all other commonly used techniques require pretreatment of samples (*6*).

The present method is submitted for use by those laboratories without expensive instrumentation, or as an alternative backup colorimetric procedure. Direct analysis of arsenic in urine can be completed in less than an hour.

Principle

The colorimetric procedure described, first used on industrial and agricultural samples, is based on liberating arsine gas (AsH_3) from the specimen (*7,8*). Potassium iodide and stannous chloride reagents reduce pentavalent arsenic to the trivalent form, which then reacts with hydrogen to produce arsine. The arsine is then directed through a solution of silver diethyldithiocarbamate in pyridine to form a soluble red compound. The intensity of the color produced is proportional to the concentration of arsenic, which can then be determined by comparison with a standard (*6,9*). Hydrogen sulfide, if produced, is removed by scrubbing the arsine with lead acetate before the color reaction. Urine can be analyzed directly, but blood, hair, nails, or other tissues must be digested with acid before the arsine generation.

Materials and Methods

Reagents

Note: All reagents should be arsenic-free or have a very low arsenic content. Check reagents for arsenic content by substituting them for urine samples in the procedure. Blanks should be included with each analytical run.

1. *Arsenic stock standard, 1.0 g/L.* Dissolve 1.32 g of arsenic trioxide in 100 mL of sodium hydroxide solution (400 g/L) and dilute to 1 L with water. Solution is stable for at least a year.
2. *Arsenic working standard, 2.5 µg/mL.* Pipet 0.50 mL of stock arsenic standard into a 200-mL volumetric flask and dilute to volume with water.
3. *Hydrochloric acid, concentrated.*
4. *Lead acetate solution.* Dissolve 10.0 g of lead acetate in 100 mL of water. Use this to impregnate glass wool that is free of heavy metals (no. 11-388; Fisher Scientific, Pittsburgh, PA). Let dry and store at room temperature.
5. *Nitric acid, concentrated.*
6. *Perchloric acid, 700 g/L, specific gravity 1.6.*
7. *Perchloric acid/nitric acid mixture.* Cautiously add 2.0 mL of nitric acid to 4.0 mL of perchloric acid and mix gently. Make up a fresh solution before use; discard the unused portion each day.
8. *Potassium iodide solution.* Dissolve 15 g of potassium iodide in 100 mL of water. Store in a brown bottle; discard when solution turns yellow.
9. *Pyridine.*
10. *Silver diethyldithiocarbamate (color reagent).* Dissolve 1.0 g of silver diethyldithiocarbamate (Fisher no. S-666) in 200 mL of pyridine and store in a brown bottle (stable for at least a year).
11. *Sodium bisulfite, granular.*
12. *Stannous chloride solution.* Dissolve 40.0 g of stannous chloride in 100 mL of concentrated hydrochloric acid and store in a brown bottle (stable for at least a year).
13. *Sulfuric acid, concentrated.*
14. *Zinc metal,* 20 mesh, arsenic-free.

Apparatus

Arsine generator with clear-seal joints (these require no grease) (Fisher no. 1-405), complete with joint clamp (Fisher no. 05-8858). This apparatus is shown in Figure 1.

Collection and Handling of Specimens

Urine: Urine is the recommended specimen for determination of arsenic because high concentrations of

---

[1] This chapter is marked "provisional," indicating that it has not met the criteria of our reviewing process. However, the method has been used extensively in the Submitter's laboratory and not only is clinically useful, but also has met standards of quality for many years.

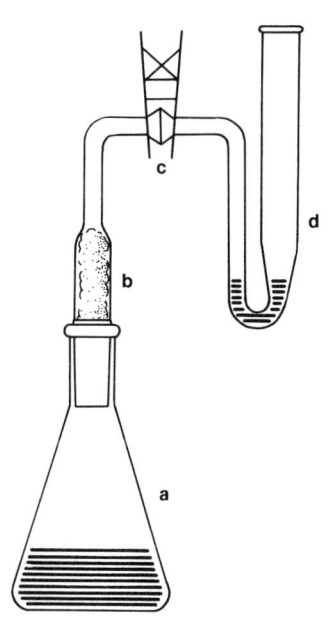

Fig. 1. Arsine generator and its components
a, flask; *b*, scrubber; *c*, clamp; *d*, absorber tube

the metal persist as long as a week after acute intoxication and as long as a month in chronic exposure *(1)*. Collect 24-h urine specimens in acid-washed polyethylene or polypropylene containers. No preservative is necessary for arsenic or other heavy metals under study. Mix the urine well, record the 24-h volume, and save 200 mL for analysis.

Blood: Collect 20 mL of whole blood into heparinized blood-collection tubes.

Stomach contents: Place in a closed polyethylene container enough stomach washing or vomitus to obtain at least 50 mL for analysis. If tissue is used, keep 50 g of tissue or other biological material refrigerated in protective containers.

Hair or nails: Samples of 1.0 to 50 g of hair or nails may be analyzed. Before digestion (see below) remove extraneous materials by washing twice with ether, dry, and record the weight.

Note: Arsenic can be detected in hair next to the root about two to three weeks after ingestion. Analysis of pubic hair is recommended for examining long-term chronic cases. Clippings from toenails may reflect exposure up to six months previously *(1)*.

Procedures

Note: 50-mL aliquots of urine, acid digests, standard, and blank are treated alike in the arsine generator. Urine is analyzed directly without digestion.

Digestion of organic material (10)

1. Place 20 mL of blood, 50 mL of stomach washings or vomitus, 50 g of macerated tissue, or as much as 50 g of hair or nails in a 300-mL Kjeldahl digestion flask.

2. Add an equal volume of concentrated nitric acid to blood, hair, nails, vomitus, or tissue; add 10 mL of the acid to 50 mL of stomach washings.

3. Add 5.0 mL of concentrated sulfuric acid and three arsenic-free glass beads. *Under a hood,* heat the mixture over a low flame until dense, white fumes evolve and the material begins to darken. Proceed with caution to prevent charring. Remove from the flame and add dropwise 1.0 mL of fresh perchloric acid/nitric acid mixture until the digest turns a clear, pale yellow.

4. Resume heating with care and repeat the addition of perchloric acid/nitric acid until the digest remains clear or faintly yellow and does not darken on further heating. Continue heating until all dense, white fumes are evolved.

5. Cool and transfer to an Erlenmeyer flask with several 5.0-mL rinses of water. Remove the remaining nitric and perchloric acids in this mixture by adding 100 mg of sodium bisulfite and boiling for 5 min until the white fumes of sulfur trioxide appear.

6. After cooling, transfer all of the sample to a 50-mL volumetric flask and dilute to volume with water.

Arsenic determination

1. Put 50 mL of urine or digested material into a labeled arsine-generator flask (see Figure 1). Put 2.0 mL of arsenic working standard plus 48 mL of water into a similar flask, and 50 mL of water into a third flask for the reagent blank.

2. Add 5 mL of concentrated hydrochloric acid and 2.0 mL of potassium iodide to each flask; mix. Add 0.40 mL of stannous chloride to each flask, mix by swirling, and let stand at room temperature for 15 min.

3. Fill the scrubber with glass wool previously treated with lead acetate. Add an additional four drops of lead acetate solution to this material, then join and clamp the scrubber to the absorber tube.

4. Place all units in the hood and add 3.0 mL of silver diethyldithiocarbamate reagent to each absorber tube. Add 3.0 g of zinc metal to a labeled flask and immediately insert the scrubber-absorber assembly. Proceed to the next flask until all have been processed.

Note: Gas evolution should begin immediately as noted by steady bubbling in the absorber tube. If not, check all joints for leaks.

5. When arsine evolution is completed (30 to 45 min), rinse the walls of the absorber tube by swirling, and transfer the silver diethyldithiocarbamate solution to cuvets. Measure absorbance of unknown and standard against the blank at 540 nm. The color is stable for 3 h.

Note: When the absorbance exceeds the limits of linearity, the sample may be diluted with unreacted color reagent, and the new absorbance reading corrected by multiplying by the dilution factor.

Quality Control

Urine Chemistry Control, Level II (Fisher Diagnostics, Orangeburg, NY), contains relatively high concentrations of arsenic and is used as a control. Make several dilutions of it to prepare controls at several concentrations. Another urine control containing arsenic is also available (UR-Sure; Hyland Laboratories, Costa Mesa, CA).

Calculations

Urine

(A unk/A std) × 5.0 × (24-h vol, mL/50) = arsenic, μg/24 h

or: (A unk/A std) × 0.10 × (24-h vol, mL/24-h vol, L) = arsenic, μg/L

Digested material

(A unk/A std) × 5.0 = μg of arsenic per 50 mL of digest

Note: For fluids, report results per milliliter of specimen; divide calculated results for 50 mL of digest by the volume of unknown used. For solids, report results per gram of specimen; divide the results for the 50 mL of digest by the weight of the sample used. For hydrated specimens (e.g., tissues), report results in terms of wet weight of sample.

Results and Discussion

Reference Values

The presence of arsenic in urine or blood is considered evidence of relatively recent absorption of this metal (10). Reference values used by the Submitter are shown in Table 1 and compared with other reported values. Bakerman (1) also reported urinary arsenic as follows: asymptomatic, up to 20 µg/L; high arsenic diet (seafood), up to 100 µg/L.

Table 1. Reference Values for Arsenic

| Concn, µg/L || Concn, µg/g, in |
Urine	Blood	hair or nails
≤ 28[a]	≤ 60[a]	≤ 3.0[a]
≤ 20 (1)	30-70 (3)	≤ 3.0 (1)
≤ 100 (2)	≤ 200 (2)	0.2 - 0.6 (3)
≤ 200 (3)	60-200 (10)	

[a] Values from the Submitter's laboratory. Other values are from references cited in parentheses.

Within-run precision of the method was determined with two urine pools obtained commercially (Fisher Diagnostics). Repetitive assays (n = 15) on these samples at two concentrations gave the following results: 169 µg/L (SD 9), CV 5.2%, and 308 µg/L (SD 14), CV 4.2%. The standard curve for the procedure is linear up to at least 300 µg of arsenic per liter of urine, as determined with dilutions of a urine control. Analytical recovery, determined by adding several concentrations of arsenic standards to pooled urine and analyzing by the present method, ranged from 91 to 105% (Table 2).

Antimony released as stibine causes some interference with color development, but at 540 nm the sensitivity for antimony is about 8% of that of arsenic (7). Also, antimony reportedly is not commonly encountered in clinical toxicology specimens (10).

Biological Considerations

Arsenic, despite its reputation as a toxic metal, is essential for normal biological functions at 30-50 ng/g (11). In persons ingesting seafood diets, the organo-arsenic from marine animals is reportedly quickly excreted in the urine without change in chemical form (6).

Arsenic has a high affinity for the keratin of hair and nails. The earliest at which arsenic can be detected in emerging hair is about two weeks after ingestion. Transverse white bands about 1 mm wide may appear across nail beds about two months after arsenic exposure (1). In addition to other major organ systems, arsenic localizes in bone four weeks after exposure. Elimination of arsenic is primarily through excretion by the kidneys, which may begin within 2 h and last up to 10 days after a single exposure.

Table 2. Analytical Recovery of Arsenic Added to Pooled Urine

| Added | Found | Recovery, % |
µg/L	µg/L	
20	18.2	91
50	47	94
100	105	105
200	192	96

References

1. Bakerman S. Metal poisoning: The laboratory detection of lead, arsenic and mercury. *Lab Manage* **21**, 13-17 (1983).
2. Brandenberger H. In *Clinical Biochemistry, Principles and Methods*, **2**, CH Curtis, M Roth, Eds., Walter de Gruyter, New York, NY, 1974, pp 1584-1603.
3. Howanitz JH, Howanitz PJ. Heavy metals. In *Clinical Diagnosis and Management by Laboratory Methods*, 16th ed., JB Henry, Ed., WB Saunders Co., Philadelphia, PA, 1979, pp 512-515.
4. Roddy TC, Wallace SM. Determination of arsenic in urine. *Am J Clin Pathol* **36**, 373-375 (1961).
5. Ratliff CR, Hall FF, Culp TW. The colorimetric determination of arsenic in biological materials. *Clin Chem* **18**, 717 (1972). Abstract.
6. Lauwerys RR, Buchet JP, Roels H. The determination of trace levels of arsenic in human biological materials. *Arch Toxicol* **41**, 238-247 (1979).
7. Liederman D, Bowen JE, Milner OJ. Determination of arsenic in petroleum stocks and catalysts by evolution as arsine. *Anal Chem* **31**, 2052-2055 (1959).
8. Horwitz W. (Ed.) *Official Methods of Analysis*, 11th ed., Association of Official Analytical Chemists, Washington, DC, 1970, pp 399-402.
9. Technical Data Bulletin no. 142, Fisher Scientific, Pittsburgh, PA 15219.
10. Leifheit HC. Arsenic in biological materials. *Stand Methods Clin Chem* **3**, 23-34 (1961).
11. Uthus EO, Collings ME, Nielson FH. Determination of total arsenic in biological samples by arsine generation and atomic absorption spectrometry. *Anal Chem* **53**, 2221-2224 (1981).

Barbiturates by Spectrophotometry

Submitters: James E. Love, Jr., and John A. Lott, Department of Pathology, The Ohio State University, Columbus, OH

Evaluators: Larry A. Broussard and Lynne Selby, Medical Laboratory Associates, Birmingham, AL

Introduction

Barbiturates are widely prescribed as sedatives, tranquilizers, and hypnotics; they are prepared by condensing urea or thiourea with a dicarboxylic acid. All are related to barbituric acid, which was first prepared in 1853 from urea and malonic acid. More than 30 different barbiturates have been used medicinally (1); at present, only five or six are in common use.

The barbiturates depress the central nervous system. Of those in current use, only phenobarbital, the most widely used barbiturate, has an anticonvulsant effect. Phenobarbital has been used to treat chronic cholestasis (2) and to induce glucuronidation of bilirubin in neonates. The drug induces the metabolism and elimination of a number of drugs such as phenytoin, prednisone, and possibly digitoxin (2). Phenobarbital exacerbates attacks of porphyria, and tends to increase alkaline phosphatase in serum of affected patients.

Chemical dependence develops after long usage of any of the barbiturates; an addicted individual can tolerate much larger doses. Sudden cessation of a barbiturate after long-time usage commonly precipitates a grand mal seizure.

The half-lives and therapeutic and toxic concentrations of the six most commonly used barbiturates are given in Table 1. The short-acting barbiturates, such as thiopental, are also the most sedating, and overdoses of short-acting barbiturates are more likely to be lethal than long-acting barbiturates such as phenobarbital. In overdose and poisoning cases, the barbiturates can produce states of consciousness ranging from drowsiness to coma. In fatal cases, the cause of death is usually respiratory arrest. Alcohol potentiates the depressant effect of barbiturates. Treatment of overdoses always involves supportive therapy. Dialysis, forced diuresis, or both, is of value in treating phenobarbital and thiopental overdoses; however, these measures are ineffective with the other barbiturates.

Phenobarbital is excreted by the kidneys, and about 30% of the dose appears unchanged in urine. Hydroxylation and glucuronidation of the drug occur in the liver.

Principle

The spectrophotometric method for barbiturates is based on the change of absorbance at 260 nm of the barbituric acid derivative when the pH is altered from 13 to 10. If the identity of the barbiturate is known, the concentration of the barbiturate can be determined; otherwise, the test is qualitative. The barbiturates are extracted from body fluids with $CHCl_3$, which is then extracted with dilute NaOH; aliquots of the alkaline extract at pH 10 and pH 13 are analyzed by spectrophotometry.

Table 1. Data on Commonly Prescribed Barbiturates

Drug	Half-life, h (reference)	Therapeutic Concn in serum, mg/L (ref.)	Toxic	Therapeutic use	Typical dose as hypnotic/sedative, mg[a]
Amobarbital	16-40 (3)	5-8 (4)	over 30 (4)	Hypnotic, sedative	65-200
			over 47 (7)		15-300
Pentobarbital	15-50[b] (3, 6)	1-4 (4)	over 5 (4)	Hypnotic, sedative	100
			over 20 (7)		40-120
Phenobarbital	53-118 (3)	15-25[c] (2)	over 40 (5)	Hypnotic, sedative, anticonvulsant	100-300
			over 65 (7)		30-120
					50-100
Secobarbital	15-40 (3)	3-5 (4)	over 5 (4)	Hypnotic, sedative	100
			over 25 (7)		50-100
Thiopental	3-8 (6)	—	—	Anesthetic	50-70 as intravenous anesthetic

[a] In adults (from reference 6). [b] Dose dependent. [c] As anticonvulsant.

Materials and Methods

Reagents

Use analytical reagent-grade chemicals and distilled water throughout.

1. *Ammonium chloride, 3.0 mol/L.* Dissolve 16 g of NH_4Cl in enough water to make 100 mL of solution.

2. *Chloroform.* Spectral grade is preferred; however, analytical reagent grade is satisfactory (e.g., from Mallinckrodt, Inc., Paris, KY 40361).

3. *Hydrochloric acid, 1 mol/L.* Dilute 8.3 mL of concd. HCl with enough water to make 100 mL.

4. *Sodium hydroxide, 0.45 mol/L.* Prepare 12.5 mol/L by dissolving 50 g of NaOH in enough water to make 100 mL of solution. Mix well, and store in a Pyrex or plastic container with a plastic or rubber closure. Prepare 0.45 mol/L NaOH solution by diluting 3.6 mL of the 12.5 mol/L NaOH solution to 100 mL with water.

5. *Stock sodium phenobarbital standard, 1 g/L.* Use a volumetric flask, and dissolve 100 mg of sodium phenobarbital in enough 0.45 mol/L NaOH to make 100 mL of solution. The stock sodium phenobarbital standard is stable for at least one year at 4 °C. Stock standards of other barbiturates can be prepared the same way.

6. *Working sodium phenobarbital standards.* Prepare 5, 10, 20, and 40 mg/L working standards by diluting 0.5, 1.0, 2.0, and 4.0 of the stock standard to 100 mL with 0.45 mol/L NaOH. Sodium phenobarbital working standards are stable for a least one year at 4 °C. Discard if any particulate matter is present.

7. Filter paper, 9 cm diameter (no. 41 H; Whatman, Inc., Clifton, NJ 07014).

8. *Controls.* Use commercially available controls with barbiturate concentrations in the therapeutic and toxic concentration ranges, or supplement pooled patients' serum with sodium phenobarbital and freeze in aliquots (2-7).

Instrument and Equipment

1. *Spectrophotometer and cuvets.* The spectrophotometer must be capable of measuring absorbance between 230 and 280 nm. A scanning spectrophotometer facilitates preparation of the absorption spectrum; however, a single-beam, nonscanning spectrophotometer is satisfactory. The wavelength calibration, absorbance accuracy, and freedom from stray light of the spectrophotometer should be confirmed as described elsewhere (8). Quartz or silica cuvets must be used, because plastic and ordinary glass cuvets are opaque to light below 260 nm.

2. *Mechanical shaker.* A shaker that can hold 50-mL polypropylene centrifuge tubes is a convenience but not a necessity.

3. *Polypropylene centrifuge tubes with tight-fitting lids.* We used "50-mL" tubes (cat. no. 25330-50; Corning Medical, Medfield, MA 02052) having a 60-mL capacity and tested by the manufacturer to be resistant to $CHCl_3$. Some plastic centrifuge tubes have glued-in lids; the $CHCl_3$ could dissolve the glue and cause the loss and (or) contamination of the extract. Separatory funnels can be used, but we found them to be difficult to handle. $CHCl_3$ tends to dissolve the stopcock grease, which may interfere with the results.

Procedure

1. Label an appropriate number of 50-mL centrifuge tubes as standards, specimens, controls, or blank (water). Pipet 3 mL of standard, specimen, control, or water into the proper tube. Add 0.15 mL of 1 mol/L HCl to the standards only. Add 50 mL of $CHCl_3$ to every tube, stopper tightly, and shake vigorously (four strokes per second) for 5 min.

2. Allow the phases to separate; remove the upper aqueous phase by aspiration, and discard it.

3. Filter the $CHCl_3$ layer through Whatman no. 41 H paper, and pipet 40 mL of the filtrate into another labeled 50-mL centrifuge tube.

4. Add 5 mL of 0.45 mol/L NaOH to the filtered $CHCl_3$ solution, and shake for 5 min. Allow the phases to separate.

5. Remove about 4 mL of the (upper) pH 13 aqueous phase from step 4, and centrifuge at 1000 × g for 10 min in labeled 13 × 100 mm glass centrifuge tubes. We suggest using tubes no. T1280-3 (American Scientific Products, McGaw Park, IL 60085).

6. Carefully pipet 3.0 mL of the pH 13 solution into a quartz or silica cuvet, and obtain the absorption spectrum between 230 and 280 nm vs the blank. With a nonscanning spectrophotometer, measurements every 5 nm suffice. Similarly scan the working standards.

7. Add 0.5 mL of 3 mol/L NH_4Cl to each cuvet to prepare the pH 10 solution. Mix, and scan again as above.

8. Examine the spectra and compare them with the spectra given in Figure 1 and the spectra you obtained for your standards. If a barbiturate is present, there should be an absorbance maximum between 252 and 255 nm and an absorbance minimum between 243 and 247 nm for the pH 13 solution. The pH 10 solution should have an absorbance maximum between 238 and 240 nm (9). If none of these conditions obtain, and the spectrum does not resemble Figure 1 or the spectra of your standards, it is unlikely that a barbiturate is present, and further calculations are pointless.

9. Calculate the concentration of the barbiturates from the absorbance (A) measurements at 260 nm:

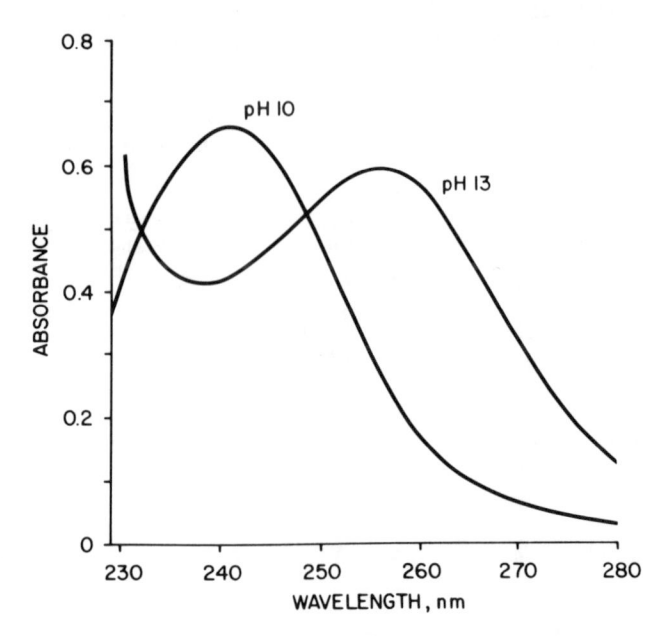

$$\Delta A = A \text{ at pH 13} - (A \text{ at pH 10} \times 1.167) \quad (1)$$

$$\text{Concn. of barb.} = \text{concn. of std.} \times (\Delta A \text{ unk.}/\Delta A \text{ std.}) \quad (2)$$

Fig. 1. Absorption spectrum of sodium phenobarbital at pH 10 and pH 13

Obtained with Model 551 (Perkin-Elmer, Norwalk, CT 06856) scanning spectrophotometer and quartz cuvets

In equation 1, 1.167 corrects for the dilution from the addition of NH$_4$Cl. Use the standard having a concentration closest to the unknown in the above calculations. The calculated concentration is valid *only* if the identity of the barbiturate is known, and if the standard compound is the same barbiturate. For phenobarbital, the method underestimates the true concentration above about 40 mg/L and overestimates the concentration below about 20 mg/L (see *Recovery studies*).

Quality Control of Procedure

At least one, and preferably two, controls should be analyzed with each group of specimens. Periodic checks of the spectrophotometer are very important, because wavelength inaccuracies and stray light will introduce serious errors. The extraction of phenobarbital is incomplete; however, with knowledge of the percent recovery, the magnitude of the error can be estimated.

Evaluation of the Procedure

Linearity. Dilutions of the stock sodium phenobarbital standard with 0.45 mol/L NaOH were prepared to obtain 10 solutions with concentrations ranging from 10 to 100 mg/L in 10 mg/L increments. These standards were analyzed in duplicate. In contrast to the serum specimens, the sodium phenobarbital standards were acidified with 0.15 mL of 1 mol/L HCl before extraction with CHCl$_3$. The difference in absorbance at 260 nm (A pH 13 − A pH 10) was proportional to concentration of sodium phenobarbital up to 100 mg/L. The regression equation was: $\Delta A = 0.00583 \times$ (concn, mg/L) − 0.0018, $r = 0.992$, standard error of slope = 0.00020. There was some scatter about the regression line as shown in Figure 2.

Recovery studies. Inter-related specimens were prepared to check the recovery of sodium phenobarbital from specimens having a constant matrix. A base pool of fresh sera with no detectable phenobarbital was supplemented with a solution of 0.5 g of sodium phenobarbital and 0.5 g of creatinine per liter of 0.45 mol/L NaOH, as follows:

Pool A: 50 mL of base pool + 10 mL of supplement solution

Pool B: 50 mL of base pool + 10 mL of NaCl, 154 mmol/L

Pools A and B were mixed in the ratios shown in Table 2. We confirmed that the specimens had been prepared properly by analyzing for creatinine. For phenobarbital, the specimens were acidified with 1 mol/L HCl to permit extraction with CHCl$_3$, and were analyzed like serum specimens, as described under *Procedure*.

At sodium phenobarbital concentrations greater than about 30 mg/L, recovery of the drug was incomplete, the percentage of recovery depending on the concentration. Correction factors could be applied, but we do not recommend this, because the factors change with concentration. When a specimen contains 40 mg of sodium phenobarbital or more per liter, the true value is about 8 mg/L greater (see Table 2). In the low therapeutic range of about 20 mg/L, the method overestimated the concentration by approximately 4 mg/L. Other barbiturates may act differently in this type of recovery study.

Reproducibility. Barbiturate-free lyophilized control serum (no. 2906-89; Fisher Scientific Co., Cincinnati, OH 45242) was supplemented with weighed sodium phenobarbital to give controls with approximately 12 and 40 mg of sodium phenobarbital per liter. These were analyzed both within-day and between-day; results are summarized in Table 3.

Interferences. The method is free from interference from many drugs, as described by Jatlow (*10*). He examined analgesics, anticoagulants, diuretics, etc., and found interferences only for *p*-aminophenol, a metabolite of acetaminophen. Because the concentrations of unconjugated *p*-aminophenol in serum are usually low, interference would not be expected (*10*).

Discussion

The procedure is as simple as most colorimetric methods, and no elaborate equipment or costly reagents are required. The test is specific for barbiturates, and few interferences should be expected. An experienced analyst

Table 2. Recovery Study with Inter-Related Specimens[a]

	Specimen no.					
	1	2	3	4	5	6
Pool A, mL	5	4	3	2	1	0
Pool B, mL	0	1	2	3	4	5
Na phenobarb. concn., mg/L						
Calculated	83.3	66.6	50.0	33.3	16.7	0
Found	64.9	51.6	40.0	31.0	19.9	0
Recovery, %[b]	78	77	80	93	119	—

[a] See text for composition of pool A and pool B.
[b] (Found/calculated) × 100.

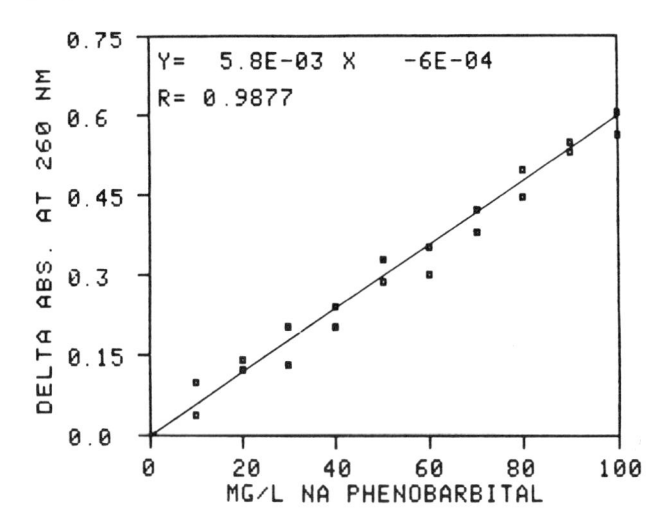

Fig. 2. Linearity plot of sodium phenobarbital standards extracted and analyzed like serum specimens

Table 3. Precision of the Method for Sodium Phenobarbital

	Concn, mg/L		
Control	Mean	SD	CV, %
Within day			
Low	10	1.4	14
High[a]	40	1.8	4.6
Between day			
Low	14	3.5	26
High	44	6.0	14

[a] n = 39. For the other assays, n = 40.

should be able to process a specimen, standard, and control in 45 min. The method is qualitative when the barbiturate is unknown; moreover, the barbiturate that is present cannot be identified from the spectrum (*11*). More definitive methods such as "high-pressure" liquid chromatography (*12*) may be necessary, particularly in the patient where poisoning with a short-acting barbiturate is suspected.

The pH of the control sera must not be above pH 7 to 7.5 after reconstitution, or extraction with $CHCl_3$ will be incomplete. Control sera with a pH below 7 are also not recommended, because interferences are more likely. Salicylic acid and other drugs will be extracted at acid pH and will shift the absorption spectrum between pH 10 and 13, leading to falsely high results for barbiturate concentrations (*10*).

We thank the staff of the Clinical Chemistry Laboratory, particularly Donna Bitzel, for their help and encouragement, and Juliene Bowen, for preparing the manuscript.

References

1. Swinyard EA. Sedatives and hypnotics. In *Remington's Pharmaceutical Sciences*, 16th ed., A Osol, GD Chase, AR Gennaro, et al., Eds., Mack Publishing Co., Easton, PA, 1980, pp 234-238.
2. Bochner F, Carruthers G, Kampmann J, et al. Phenobarbital. In *Handbook of Clinical Pharmacology*, Little, Brown and Co., Boston, MA, 1978, p 250.
3. Harvey SC. Hypnotics and sedatives. In *The Pharmacological Basis of Therapeutics*, 6th ed., A Goodman, LS Gilman, A Gilman, Eds., Macmillan Publishing Co., New York, NY, 1980, p 359.
4. Baselt RC, Cravey RH. A compendium of therapeutic and toxic concentrations of toxicologically significant drugs in biofluids. *J Anal Toxicol* **1**, 81-103 (1977).
5. Kutt H, Penry JK. Usefulness of blood levels of antiepileptic drugs. *Arch Neurol* **31**, 283-288 (1974).
6. *Drug Facts and Comparisons*, JR Boyd, Ed., JB Lippincott Co., Philadelphia, PA, 1984.
7. Spiegel HE. Barbiturates, ultraviolet spectrophotometric method. In *Selected Methods for the Small Clinical Laboratory*, W Faulkner, S Meites, Eds., American Association for Clinical Chemistry, Washington, DC, 1982, pp 109-111.
8. Lott JA. Practical problems in clinical enzymology. *Crit Rev Clin Lab Sci* **8**, 277-301 (1977).
9. Blanke RV. Analysis of drugs and toxic substances. In *Fundamentals of Clinical Chemistry*, NW Tietz, Ed., WB Saunders Co., Philadelphia, PA, 1970, p 1143.
10. Jatlow P. Ultraviolet spectrophotometric analysis of barbiturates. *Am J Clin Pathol* **59**, 167-173 (1973).
11. Goldbaum LR. Analytical determination of barbiturates. *Anal Chem* **24**, 1600-1607 (1952).
12. Gill R, Lopes AAT, Moffat AC. Analysis of barbiturates in blood by high-performance liquid chromatography. *J Chromatogr* **226**, 117-123 (1981).

Bromide in Serum by Spectrophotometry

Submitter: Charles A. Bradley, *Department of Pathology Vanderbilt University, Nashville, TN*

Evaluator: Kenneth E. Blick, *University of Oklahoma College of Medicine, Oklahoma City, OK 73190*

Introduction

Determination of bromide in blood may be required in instances of intoxication from an overdose of sedatives containing bromides. Although the availability of bromide-containing therapeutic compounds is declining, certain nerve tonics and headache remedies still contain bromide (1). Moreover, certain organic bromides, such as carbromal (a sedative) and methyl bromide (a fumigant) can also produce substantial amounts of this halide (2). Acute bromide intoxication is rare: the drug irritates the gastrointestinal tracts, making it difficult to ingest and retain toxic concentrations of bromide without vomiting. Continued interest in bromide analysis is directed primarily toward patients with chronic bromide intoxication from indiscriminate use of bromide-containing over-the-counter medications. Bromides are excreted slowly by the kidney and are therefore likely to accumulate after chronic ingestion. About 4.3% of a dose is excreted daily, corresponding to an elimination half-life of about 12 days (3).

Clinical manifestation of bromide intoxication includes fever, neurologic disturbances, skin rash, and a history of ingesting bromide-containing drugs (4). Neurologic abnormalities may include tremors and disruption of motor coordination. Chronic bromide poisoning may also be associated with increases in cerebrospinal fluid pressure, as well as increases in protein concentration in cerebrospinal fluid. Certain patients may experience mental malfunction, which can persist for some time after the drug has been eliminated from the body. Alcoholics appear to be particularly susceptible to bromide intoxication.

Distribution of bromide in the body is similar to that of chloride. Tissues do not readily distinguish between chloride and bromide, and ingestion of either halide results in the displacement of the other. The similarity of atomic structure of bromide and chloride means that many of the clinical laboratory methods for measuring chloride are subject to interference by bromide. Therefore, spuriously high concentrations of chloride in a patient raise the suspicion of bromide intoxication (5).

Principle

The method described here is essentially that of Wuth (6). Only free Br^- is measured; bromide in organic compounds will not be detected. However, ingested organic bromides are metabolized to inorganic free Br^- for subsequent quantification.

This assay utilizes the displacement of chloride from gold trichloride by the bromide anion to form gold tribromide:

$$AuCl_3 + 3\ Br^- \rightarrow AuBr_3 + 3\ Cl^-$$

The formation of $AuBr_3$ may also be accompanied by the formation of $AuBrCl_2$ and $AuBr_2Cl$. The gold bromide complex is brown, and can be quantitatively measured in a spectophotometer at 440 nm.

Materials and Methods

Collection and Handling of Specimens

No special preparation of the patient is necessary. Blood should be collected in chemically clean evacuated tubes or syringes, without anticoagulants. Hemolyzed specimens are not acceptable. Each bromide analysis requires 2 mL of serum, which should be stored refrigerated at 2-8 °C.

Reagents

1. *Trichloroacetic acid (TCA) solution:* Dissolve 10 g of TCA and 0.6 g of sodium chloride (NaCl) with reagent-grade water in a 100-mL volumetric flask; dilute to volume. This should be stable for at least 90 days when stored at room temperature in a brown glass bottle.

2. *Gold chloride solution:* Dissolve 0.5 g of $AuCl_3 \cdot HCl \cdot 3\ H_2O$ in water and dilute to 100 mL. Stored at room temperature in a brown glass bottle, the reagent should be stable for at least 90 days.

3. *Stock bromide standard:* Use 1.288 g of sodium bromide (M_r 102.90) or 1.489 g of potassium bromide (M_r 119.01). Whichever compound is used, dry at 110 °C for 12 h. The bromide (M_r 79.91) crystals are then dissolved in reagent-grade water and diluted to 250 mL; the final concentration is 4000 mg/L or 50 mmol/L. This is stable for at least six months at room temperature.

4. *Working bromide standards:* Dilute 5.0 and 10.0 mL of the stock standard to 50 mL with reagent-grade water; final bromide concentrations are 400 and 800 mg/L, respectively. These are also stable for at least six months at room temperature.

Procedure

1. Pipet 8.0 mL of the TCA solution into a 15 × 150 mm test tube.

2. Add 2.0 mL of serum and vortex-mix. Let the tubes stand for 10 min, then centrifuge at 1000 × *g*.

3. If the supernate is not perfectly clear, filter (e.g., with no. 1 filter paper; Whatman Laboratory Products, Clifton, NJ).

4. Prepare standards and a blank by pipetting 2.0 mL of the two working standards or 2.0 mL of water plus 8.0 mL

of TCA solution into labeled test tubes. These solutions will have no precipitate and thus do not need to be centrifuged or filtered.

5. Pipet 4.0-mL aliquots of the supernates from the samples, standards, and blank into test tubes, then add 1.0 mL of the gold chloride solution and vortex-mix.

6. Let the tubes stand at room temperature for 10 min, then read the absorbance of the standards and samples against the blank at 440 nm.

Calculations

The standards and samples are treated similarly so that:

$$\text{Concn of sample} = \frac{A \text{ sample}}{A \text{ standard}} \times \text{concn of standard}$$

For calculations, use the standard whose absorbance reading (A) is closest to that of the sample.

Quality Control

Because commercially available control materials do not contain bromide, each laboratory must prepare its own controls. It is desirable to prepare two serum pools, with different concentrations of either sodium or potassium bromide. Aliquots of the pools should be frozen until an assay is to be performed.

Results and Discussion

Normal concentrations of bromide in human blood average 3 to 4 mg/L (7). This method does not detect such low concentrations of bromide but will detect concentrations less than those that cause toxic symptoms to appear, e.g., 6 to 12 mmol/L (0.50 to 1.00 g/L) (8). At concentrations between 20 and 30 mmol/L (1.60 to 2.40 g/L), the patients may show psychotic behavior such as emotional outbursts and lose motor coordination. Concentrations exceeding 40 mmol/L (320 g/L) may be fatal.

As mentioned, acute intoxication with bromide is rare 9). Chronic intoxication usually takes two to four weeks to develop and is often mistaken for numerous other diseases that affect the central nervous system. Treatment of bromide intoxication involves proper hydration and the administration of chloride and (or) diuretics to promote bromide excretion. With these procedures the half-life of bromide in plasma can be reduced from 12 days to 65 h or less (10). In severe cases, hemodialysis has reduced the half-life to 30 min (11).

Note: Large quantities of bromide in the blood will be measured as chloride in the methods for chloride determinations commonly used in the routine clinical chemistry laboratory. To calculate the true concentration of chloride in a serum containing bromide, convert the bromide concentration to mmol/L [Br, mg/L × 1/80 = Br, mmol/L] and subtract from the apparent chloride concentration (12).

References

1. Howanitz JH, Howanitz PJ, Henry JB. In *Clinical Diagnosis and Management by Laboratory Methods*, JB Henry, Ed., WB Saunders Co., Philadelphia, PA, 1979, p 504.
2. Baselt RC. *Analytical Procedures for Therapeutic Drug Monitoring and Emergency Toxicology,* Biomedical Publications, Davis, CA, 1980, p 58.
3. Soremark R. The biological half-life of bromide ions in human blood. *Acta Physiol Scand* **50**, 119-123 (1960).
4. Trump DL, Hockberg MC. Bromide intoxication. *Johns Hopkins Med J* **138**, 119 (1976).
5. Wenk RE, Lustgarten JA, Pappas J, et al. Serum chloride analysis, bromide detection, and the diagnosis of bromism. *Am J Clin Pathol* **64**, 49-57 (1976).
6. Wuth O. Rational bromide treatment. *J Am Med Assoc* **88**, 2013-2018 (1927).
7. Cross JD, Smith H. Bromide in human tissue. *Forens Sci* **11**, 147-153 (1978).
8. Toro G, Ackermann PG. *Practical Clinical Chemistry,* Little, Brown and Co., Boston, MA, 1975, p 671.
9. Baselt RC. *Disposition of Toxic Drugs and Chemicals in Man,* Biomedical Publications, Davis, CA, 1982, p 86.
10. Moses H, Klawans HL. Bromide intoxication. *Handb Clin Neurol* **36**, 291-318 (1979).
11. Wieth JO, Funder J. Treatment of bromide poisoning. *Lancet* **ii**, 327-329 (1963).
12. Annino JS, Gise RW. *Clinical Chemistry Principles and Procedures,* Little, Brown and Co., Boston, MA, 1976, p 354.

Carboxyhemoglobin by Spectrophotometry

Submitter: Earle W. Holmes, *Department of Pathology, Stritch School of Medicine, Loyola University Medical Center, Maywood, IL 60153*

Evaluators: H. Patrick Covault and T. Sabapathy, *Department of Pathology, St. Francis Hospital of Evanston, Evanston, IL 60202*

Introduction

Carbon monoxide (CO) is a tasteless, odorless gas generated by the incomplete combustion of carbonaceous materials. Important sources of CO include internal combustion engines, improperly vented natural gas heaters, smoke from burning buildings, and tobacco smoke (*1*). The toxic effects of CO are due to tissue hypoxia or anoxia. The affinity of hemoglobin for CO is approximately 200-fold greater than its affinity for oxygen. As the CO content of blood increases, the amount of hemoglobin available to carry oxygen decreases, and the dissociation curve of the remaining oxyhemoglobin (HbO$_2$) is shifted such that its ability to release oxygen to the tissues is diminished. CO is frequently involved in both accidental and suicidal poisonings. The fact that 40% of the deaths by suicide in 1978 involved CO poisoning (*2*) underscores the need for the determination of this substance in the emergency toxicology laboratory.

Among the analytical methods available for the measurement of CO in tissues and biological fluids are those involving gas chromatography (*3*), gasometric techniques (*4*), and Conway microdiffusion (*5*), as well as several spectrophotometric methods in which CO is measured as carboxyhemoglobin (HbCO) (*6*). The spectrophotometric determinations have advantages over the other methods by being rapid and easy to perform, and requiring only a minimum of specialized equipment.

A spectrophotometric method for the determination of HbCO in the presence of HbO$_2$ was first presented in 1900 (*7*). Hüfner reported that the ratio of the absorbances of a mixture of HbCO and HbO$_2$ at 541 nm and 560 nm was proportional to the percentage of the hemoglobin in the mixture that was saturated with CO (%CO saturation). Over the years, this basic methodology has been modified by changing the wavelengths at which the absorbances were measured (*8*), measuring the absorbance at three or more wavelengths (*9*), or reducing the mixture of hemoglobins before measuring the absorbances (*10*). These various modifications have been aimed at increasing the sensitivity, specificity, and precision of the assay.

The method presented here is essentially that of Tietz and Fiereck (*11,12*), who determined %CO saturation by measuring the absorbances of a mixture of reduced hemoglobins at 541 and 555 nm. This method, unlike the direct spectrophotometric assay of Amenta (*9*), is not subject to interference by bilirubin and other hemoglobin derivatives (*11*). The current method is free from interference by methemoglobin, and is characterized by a standard curve that is linear throughout the analytical range. It is suitable for the rapid determination of %CO saturation in blood obtained from victims of CO poisoning.

Principle

The concentration of each component of a mixture of absorbing substances can be determined if there are distinct differences in their absorption spectra, and if the Lambert-Beer law applies to each (*13*). For a two-component system, the ratio of the absorbance of any mixture at two wavelengths (λ_1/λ_2) will have a value intermediate between the ratios of each of the pure components. This intermediate value will depend on the concentration of each of the two components (*10*).

In the method described here, a hemolysate of whole blood is treated with sodium hydrosulfite before its absorbance is measured at 541 and 555 nm. This treatment enhances the differences between the absorption spectra of HbCO and HbO$_2$ by converting the latter to deoxyhemoglobin (spectra presented in references *10-12*). In addition, methemoglobin in the specimen is converted to deoxyhemoglobin. The %CO saturation of the hemolysate is determined from the absorbance ratio (A_{541}/A_{555}) by comparison with a standard curve.

Materials and Methods

Reagents

1. *Ammonia*, 0.23 mol/L. Dilute 16 mL of concentrated NH$_4$OH (AR, 28.2% as NH$_3$) to 1 L with de-ionized water. This solution is stable for at least six months when stored tightly capped.

2. *Sodium hydrosulfite* (AR) *powder*. Store 10-mg portions of Na$_2$S$_2$O$_4$ in small, stoppered tubes at room temperature. When kept dry, the powder is stable indefinitely. *Caution:* This is a flammable solid in the presence of moisture.

3. *Carbon monoxide*, C. P. (Matheson, Joliet, IL 60434). *Caution:* This is a toxic, flammable gas.

4. *Oxygen*, 99.9% minimum purity (Matheson).

   Note: The Evaluators obtained satisfactory results with USP-grade oxygen.

5. *Nitrogen*, prepurified (Matheson).

Apparatus

1. *Spectrophotometer.* A narrow bandpass (<2 nm) spectrophotometer (Zeiss M4QIII; Carl Zeiss, Inc., Thornwood, NY 10594, or equivalent) and 1-cm glass cuvets are required for maximum analytical sensitivity.

Note: The Evaluators used a spectrophotometer equipped with automatic wavelength and absorbance calibration and automatic wavelength selection (Response; Gilford, Oberlin, OH 44074).

2 Blood-gas equilibration vessel. Blood is equilibrated with O_2, CO, and N_2 in a 50-mL hypovial containing a Teflon-covered magnetic stirring bar and capped with a rubber-septum stopper. The stopper is pierced with two 20-gauge hypodermic needles. Gas is introduced into the vial through one needle and exhausted through the other, while the blood in the vial is mixed slowly (<140 rpm) on a magnetic stirring plate.

Collection and Handling of Specimens

Collect whole blood (arterial or venous), with heparin as the anticoagulant. It is best to analyze the specimen without delay, but the blood may be stored refrigerated (tightly stoppered and protected from light) for several days before analysis. This method is not suitable for analysis of postmortem blood or specimens containing denatured hemoglobin.

Procedure

1. Collect a specimen of blood from a healthy nonsmoker for use as a control. (A suitable commercial control may be used instead, if desired.)

2. Prepare hemolysates by adding 0.1 mL of blood from the patient or the control to 25 mL of the 0.23 mol/L NH_3 solution. Mix each and let stand for at least 2 min.

3. Transfer 3 mL of each hemolysate to a glass 1-cm-square cuvet. Transfer 3 mL of 0.23 mol/L NH_3 solution to a third cuvet to serve as a blank.

4. Add 10 mg of sodium hydrosulfite to each cuvet, cover with Parafilm, and mix by gentle inversion. The addition of the reducing agent to multiple cuvets should be carried out at 1- to 2-min intervals so that the absorbances of each can be determined exactly 5 min later.

5. Measure the absorbance of each reduced hemolysate at 541 and 555 nm, relative to the blank, exactly 5 min after the addition of the hydrosulfite.

Note: If the hemoglobin content of the sample is extremely high or low, the initial dilution should be adjusted so that the absorbance of the hemolysate at 541 is in the range of 0.2 to 0.5.

6. Calculate the absorbance ratio (A_{541}/A_{555}) for each specimen and determine the %CO saturation by interpolation from the standard curve.

Note: The Evaluators prefer to express their results in SI units, in which the proportion of HbCO is expressed as a fraction. Multiply %CO saturation units by 0.01 to convert them to this expression.

Preparation of the Standard Curve

Standards are analyzed in triplicate exactly as described above.

1. Collect 10-mL of heparinized blood from a nonsmoker and transfer 4-mL aliquots to each of two gas-equilibration vessels.

2. Equilibrate one aliquot with CO by delivering a steady stream of gas through the inlet needle (a flow rate of 300 mL/min is sufficient). After 15 min, shut off the gas supply and stir the blood for an additional 15 min. Immediately analyze samples of this equilibrated blood to establish the absorbance ratio of a specimen exhibiting 100% CO saturation.

3. Treat the remainder of this specimen with nitrogen for 5 min (to remove physically dissolved CO), cap it tightly, and set aside.

4. Using the protocol described in step 2, equilibrate a second aliquot of blood with oxygen and calculate its absorbance ratio. The observed ratio constitutes that expected in a specimen exhibiting 0% CO saturation.

5. Plot the average absorbance ratios (ordinate) of the two standards against %CO saturation and draw a line connecting the two points (Figure 1).

6. Analyze the nitrogen-treated blood (from step 3) and determine its exact %CO saturation by using the two-point standard curve; the result will be less than 100% because a small amount of CO will dissociate from the hemoglobin during the treatment with nitrogen. Mix this blood with the 0% standard in different proportions to prepare two or more intermediate standards. When plotted against the %CO saturation expected (based on the absorbance ratios of the standards prepared in steps 4 and 6 and the relative proportion of each in the mixtures), the absorbance ratios of the intermediate points should fall on the standard curve.

Note: The standard curve obtained by the Evaluators for 0, 33, 50, 66, and 100% standards is superimposable on the curve shown in Figure 1.

A separate standard curve must be prepared for each spectrophotometer used in the analysis. The assay should be restandardized periodically as dictated by various accrediting agencies, and after maintenance of the spectrophotometer.

Quality Control

The average absorbance ratios observed for the 0 and 100% standards in the course of periodic restandardization of the assay by the Submitter and the Evaluators are shown in Table 1A. Tietz and Fiereck (*11*) reported absorbance ratios for the 0 and 100% standards of 0.825 ± 0.005 and 1.223 ± 0.005, respectively (mean ± SD). When the absorbance ratios of the standards deviate widely from these average values, it may indicate the

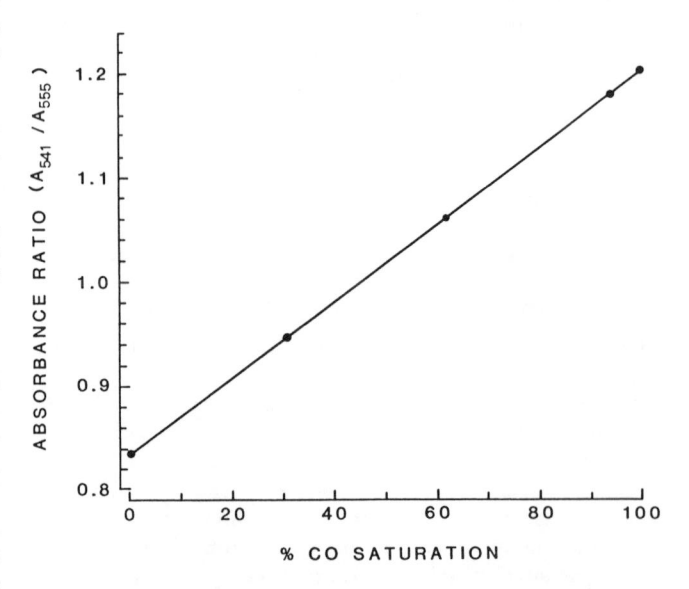

Fig. 1. Standard curve for the HbCO assay

Standards were prepared and assayed in triplicate as described in *Procedure*. The nitrogen-treated 100% standard had a CO saturation of 94%. The two intermediate standards had expected values of 62 and 31%, in excellent agreement with the values calculated from their absorbance ratios with the two-point standard curve

Table 1. Precision of the Spectrophotometric Assay for Carboxyhemoglobin

		Absorbance ratio		%CO saturation		
Specimen	n	Mean	SD	Mean	SD	CV, %
A. Successive standard curves[a]						
S: 0% Std.	6	0.831	0.008			1.0
100% Std.	6	1.249	0.026			2.08
E: 0% Std.	5	0.837	0.001			0.07
100% Std.	5	1.200	0.007			0.56
B. Within-day precision						
S: 0% Std.	10	0.837	0.004			0.50
100% Std.	10	1.210	0.007			0.60
E: Quantra I	20			12.54	0.05	0.39
C. Day-to-day precision						
S: Quantra I	15			11.4	1.21	10.6
Quantra III	15			37.1	0.85	2.3
E: Quantra I	20			12.46	0.12	0.94

[a] Based on results obtained over a three-year period by the Submitter (S) and over a one-month period by the Evaluators (E).

presence of an interfering substance in the standard, inadequate saturation of the standards with O_2 or CO, or a problem with the calibration of the spectrophotometer. The day-to-day performance of the assay may be assessed in several ways. Blood from apparently normal, nonsmoking individuals may be assayed as controls along with specimens from patients. Recently, commercial control materials containing HbCO have become available. One of these (Quantra Plus; American Dade, Miami, FL 33152) has been tested and appears to be a satisfactory control material for use with this test. The spectrophotometer used for the analysis should be subjected to routine quality-control procedures, including checks of the accuracy of the wavelength and absorbance calibrations as well as for linearity and stray light. This will require use of appropriate filters or liquid reference materials.

Results and Discussion

Analytical Variables

The present method has been widely recommended (6,12,14) for determining HbCO in an emergency toxicology setting. The reagents are stable, inexpensive, and easy to prepare, and the apparatus required is available in most laboratories. Once a standard curve has been prepared, a test result can be obtained in 10 to 15 min. The precision of the assay is largely independent of the precision of the sample dilution because absorbance ratios rather than absolute values are used in the calculation. One critical aspect of the assay is the duration of the sodium hydrosulfite treatment (see reference 11 for a further discussion of this point). It is also important that the accuracy of the wavelength and absorbance calibrations of the spectrophotometer be maintained to ensure the validity of the standard curve over an extended period.

Specificity. The method is free from interference by methemoglobin and bilirubin, but sulfhemoglobin is known to be a source of interference. However, this pigment is generally assumed to be absent from specimens submitted for HbCO determinations. The presence of sulfhemoglobin or other abnormal pigments in a specimen may be detected by recording the complete absorption spectra of the hemolysate before and after reduction. Sulfhemoglobin, if present, will have an absorption maximum at about 620 nm that is not affected by reduction with sodium hydrosulfite. Alternative methods should be used to determine CO in specimens obtained postmortem (5,16), because these are more likely to contain interfering pigments.

Precision, analytical recovery, and sensitivity. The results of precision studies are shown in Table 1, B and C. The day-to-day CV of 2.3% observed at an average %CO saturation of 37 is similar to the value reported by Tietz and Fiereck (11) for a sample with a comparable %CO saturation. The precision of the present method also compares favorably with that of several other manual spectrophotometric HbCO assays (8,11).

Note: The Evaluators performed the assay with greater precision than did the Submitter. In particular, there is an impressive difference between the two laboratories in day-to-day precision when the Quantra I control was used. This difference is most likely due to the fact that the Evaluators used a spectrophotometer that could be set up more reproducibly from day to day (see *Apparatus*).

Studies carried out by the Evaluators (Table 2) demonstrated a good recovery of HbCO throughout the range of saturations in which the characteristic clinical symptoms of CO poisoning are first manifest.

Table 2. Analytical Recovery Study[a]

%CO saturation		% recovery
Predicted	Observed	
15.5	15.3	98.7
18.0	17.5	97.2
21.0	21.0	100.0
		Mean 98.6

[a] Commercial control materials were mixed in different proportions to prepare mixtures with three different %CO saturations. Each mixture was assayed in duplicate and the average analytical recovery was calculated.

Based on the mean and SD for the 0% standard (Table 1B), the detection limit for the assay (mean result for the zero standard + 2.6 SD) is between 1 and 5% CO saturation.

Note: The Evaluators observed the lower detection limit, given the increased precision of their assay.

Correlation. The present method has already been compared with two other manual spectrophotometric assays for HbCO (11). Figure 2 shows the results of a comparison between the present method and the IL 282 Co-Oximeter (Instrumentation Laboratory, Inc., Lexington, MA 02173). Those by the present method averaged about 2% lower than those determined with the Co-Oximeter.

Note: The Evaluators also found a small negative bias in their correlation study.

The bias between the methods is not likely to influence the interpretation of %CO saturation results in CO poisoning. The correlation between the results of the two methods was excellent.

Reference Values

Healthy nonsmokers living in environments where the exposure to CO is minimal may be expected to have CO saturations in the range of 0.5 to 2.0% (11). The presence

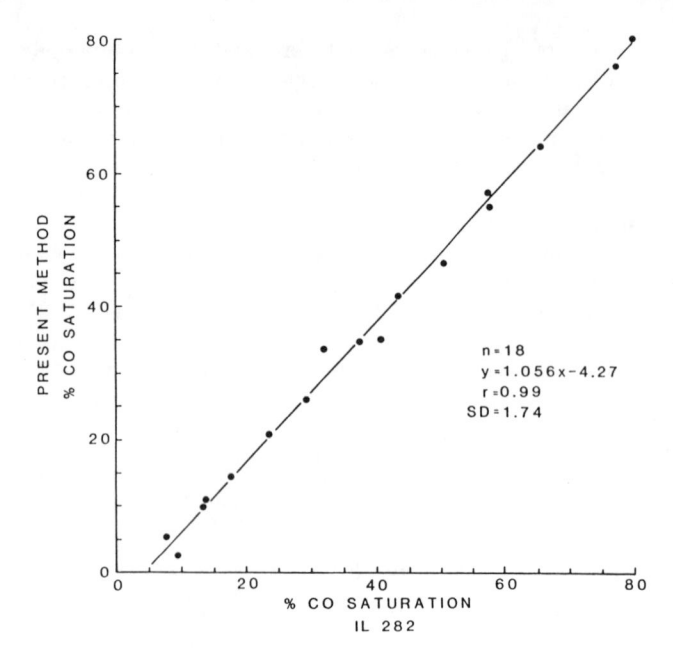

Fig. 2. Comparison of results by the manual method with those by the IL 282 Co-Oximeter

Pooled heparinized blood was tonometered with CO and assayed by both methods. The IL 282 method is based on a direct spectrophotometric analysis of hemoglobins at four wavelengths. With the IL 282, the final %CO saturation is automatically calculated with a series of simultaneous equations. The manufacturer claims that this instrument has a precision of 0.5% and an accuracy of better than 1% throughout the analytical range (0-100% CO saturation). *Solid line:* y = x

of HbCO in these individuals is from the production of CO in the body during heme catabolism. Nonsmokers living in urban environments have CO saturations of 5% or less, whereas individuals chronically exposed to automobile exhaust in the workplace (e.g., garage workers, cab drivers, traffic police) may have CO saturations in the range of 3 to 15% (*1*). Smokers may have CO saturations that range from 4 to 20%, depending on their smoking history (*1,11,14*).

Deficiencies in visual acuity and performance in certain psychological tests have been documented in laboratory studies of individuals with CO saturation of no more than 10% (*1*). Mild physical symptoms of CO poisoning such as slight headache and slight dyspnea on exertion may occur at CO saturations of 10 to 15% (*15*). At saturations of 20 to 30%, the major symptoms of CO poisoning occur: severe headache, irritability, ready fatigue, and impaired judgement (*11*). Saturations of 60 to 70% are associated with loss of consciousness, respiratory failure, and death, unless promptly treated, and exposures resulting in 80% or more CO saturation are rapidly fatal (*11*). The toxic effects associated with a given percentage of saturation depend on the general condition of the patient, the pre-existing concentration of blood hemoglobin, and the duration of the exposure to the gas (*15*). The significance of a particular percentage saturation in a poisoned patient is best judged in light of the elimination half-life of CO, which is approximately 4 h in a person breathing uncontaminated atmospheric air (*15*) and ranges from 1 to 2 h in a person treated with 100% oxygen (*1*).

Dorothy Gargano is gratefully acknowledged for her help in preparing this manuscript.

References

1. Dreisbach RH. *Handbook of Poisoning*, 10th ed., Lange Medical Publications, Los Altos, CA, 1980, pp 254-258.
2. Poklis A, Pesce AJ. Toxicology. In *Clinical Chemistry, Theory, Analysis, and Correlation*, LA Kaplan, AJ Pesce, Eds., CV Mosby Co., St. Louis, MO, 1984, p 903.
3. Collison HA, Rodkey FL, O'Neal JD. Determination of carbon monoxide in blood by gas chromatography. *Clin Chem* 14, 162-171 (1968).
4. Van Slyke DD, Robscheit-Robbins FS. The gasometric determination of small amounts of carbon monoxide in blood, and its application to blood volume studies. *J Biol Chem* 72, 39-50 (1927).
5. Feldstein M, Klendshoj N. The determination of volatile substances by microdiffusion analysis. *J Forens Sci* 2, 39-58 (1957).
6. Makarem A. Hemoglobins, myoglobins, and haptoglobins. In *Clinical Chemistry, Principles and Technics*, 2nd ed., RJ Henry, DC Cannon, JW Winkleman, Eds., Harper and Row, Hagerstown, MD, 1974, p 2245.
7. Hüfner G. Uber die gleichzeitige quantitative Bestimmung zweier Farbstoffe im Blute mit Hülfe des Spectrophotometers. *Arch Anat Physiol, Physiol Abt,* 39, 63 (1900).
8. Heilmeyer L. *Spectrophotometry in Medicine*, pt. 2, London, 1943, pp 65-94.
9. Amenta JS. The spectrophotometric determination of carbon monoxide in blood. *Stand Methods Clin Chem* 4, 31-38 (1963).
10. Klendshoj NC, Feldstein M, Sprague AL. The spectrophotometric determination of carbon monoxide. *J Biol Chem* 183, 297-303 (1950).
11. Tietz NW, Fiereck EA. The spectrophotometric measurement of carboxyhemoglobin. *Ann Clin Lab Sci* 3, 36-42 (1973).
12. Blanke RV. Analysis of drugs and toxic substances. In *Fundamentals of Clinical Chemistry*, 2nd ed., NW Tietz, Ed., WB Saunders Co., Philadelphia, PA, 1976, pp 1103-1109.
13. Van Kampen EJ, Zilstra WG. Determination of hemoglobin and its derivatives. *Adv Clin Chem* 8, 141-187 (1965).
14. Bauer JD. *Clinical Laboratory Methods*, CV Mosby Co., St. Louis, MO, 1982, p 42.
15. Bauer JD. Hemoglobin, porphyrin and iron metabolism *Op. cit.* (ref. 2), p 632.
16. Hayashi T, Nanikawa R. Further study on spectrophotometric determination of CO-Hb in post-mortem blood. *Forens Sci* 11, 127-134 (1978).

Cyanide and Thiocyanate by Microdiffusion and Spectrophotometry

Submitters: Horace E. Hamilton, Ernest W. Street, Mona Beckman Royder, and Keith Adams, *Harris Medical Laboratory, Fort Worth, TX 76113*

Evaluators: F. Leland McClure and Gaylon A. Peyton, *Texas College of Osteopathic Medicine, Fort Worth, TX*

Introduction

Any analytical method purported to support the emergency diagnosis and treatment of cyanide poisoning must provide results on a timely basis because this toxicant acts rapidly. Though it has been suggested (1) that cyanide analyses are useful only for documentation, the prepared laboratory can provide analytical results within a time that will allow effective therapy with specific antidotes; contrary to common belief, survival for several hours after ingestions of even supralethal amounts of cyanide, particularly with supportive treatment, is not uncommon (2,3). The laboratory should also be able to provide rapid and reliable determination of the cyanide metabolite, thiocyanate. Whereas cyanide in whole blood is relatively stable for several days, even at ambient temperature, because of the tight binding of cyanhemoglobin, cyanide in plasma is rapidly converted to thiocyanate (4). Hence, whereas whole blood or gastric specimens may be analyzed for cyanide, one should analyze plasma, serum, and urine specimens for thiocyanate because their cyanide content may at most be only moderately increased, even in acute poisonings. Whole blood is, of course, the specimen of choice for clinical evaluation.

The numerous methods for the determination of cyanide include the use of ultraviolet spectrophotometry, fluorometry, atomic absorption spectrophotometry, potentiometry, gas chromatography, mass spectrometry, and colorimetry with various chromogens. To isolate and concentrate the cyanide ions before the detection steps, analysts commonly use aeration, steam distillation, and microdiffusion. Bark and Higson (5), reviewing the methods available for estimating small amounts of cyanide, suggested that colorimetric methods were superior, the colorimetric methods based upon the König synthesis of pyridine dyestuffs (6) being the most suitable. Pettigrew and Fell (4) reviewed cyanide determinations based on modifications of the König synthesis, and described simplified colorimetric procedures for the routine direct determination of thiocyanate (4) or for the determination of cyanide after microdiffusion (7). Here we describe modifications of Pettigrew and Fell's procedures that significantly decrease analysis time. With this procedure cyanide concentration can be reported within 40 min of receipt of specimen, as compared with about 2.5 h by the unmodified procedure. Within the past year, the described method has, in the Submitters' laboratory, contributed to the survival of two patients who ingested potentially lethal amounts of potassium cyanide in adulterated antibiotic capsules (8).

Principle

In this procedure cyanogen bromide reacts with pyridine/p-phenylenediamine to produce a colored complex. Both thiocyanate and cyanide will undergo the following reactions:

(1a) $KSCN + 4 Br_2 + 4 H_2O \rightarrow CNBr + 6 HBr + H_2SO_4 + KBr$

(1b) $HCN + Br_2 \rightarrow CNBr + HBr$

(2) $CNBr + $ pyridine/p-phenylenediamine $\rightarrow$ pyridine dye

Materials and Methods

Reagents

1. *Bromine water, saturated.*

2. *Arsenous oxide solution (0.1 mol/L), pH 7.6.* Dissolve 2.0 g of As_2O_3 in 100 mL of 0.1 mol/L sodium hydroxide. As_2O_3 is sparingly soluble; heat the alkali solution briefly in a boiling water bath (*under a fume hood: As_2O_3 is toxic!*) and shake vigorously and frequently. When the solution cools to room temperature, adjust the pH to 7.6 ± 0.4 with dropwise addition of concentrated hydrochloric acid. Stable for one year when refrigerated.

3. *Phenylenediamine, 2.00 g/L (18.5 mmol/L) in 0.5 mol/L hydrochloric acid:* Stable for three months when protected from light (in an amber bottle) and refrigerated.

4. *Pyridine reagent*: Mix 30 mL of pyridine, 5 mL of concentrated hydrochloric acid, and 20 mL of de-ionized water. Stable for at least three months when stored refrigerated.

> *Note*: It is expedient to keep reagents 2-4 together in the refrigerator in a small box labeled "Cyanide Assay."

5. *Chromogenic reagent*: Combine three volumes of pyridine reagent (reagent 4) with one volume of phenylenediamine reagent (reagent 3). Prepare fresh, within 2 h of analyses. (It is convenient to prepare this reagent during the diffusion step of the procedure.)

6. *Hydrochloric acid, 1 mol/L.*

7. *Trichloroacetic acid, 100 g/L (0.61 mol/L).* (Required for the thiocyanate assay, but not for the cyanide assay.)

8. *Sodium hydroxide, 0.1 mol/L.* (Required for the cyanide assay, but not for the thiocyanate assay.)

9. *Sulfuric acid, 10 mol/L.* (Required for the cyanide assay, but not for the thiocyanate assay.) To approximately 20 mL of de-ionized water, slowly add 27.8 mL of concentrated sulfuric acid, and carefully mix. When cooled

to ambient temperature, dilute to 50 mL with de-ionized water.

10. *Cyanide stock standard, 9.6 mmol/L (250 mg/L)*. Dissolve 62.5 mg of potassium cyanide in 50 mL of 0.1 mol/L sodium hydroxide. Stable at least one year when stored refrigerated.

11. *Blood cyanide standards*. Mix 200 µL of cyanide stock standard with 1.8 mL of "normal blood," preferably pooled from random blood specimens from several individuals not exposed to cyanide. Mix 100 and 300 µL of this intermediate standard with 2.5 and 2.7 mL of normal blood, for cyanide standards of 40 and 100 µmol/L, respectively (adjusted for mean blood cyanide concentration of 2.7 µmol/L).

12. *Thiocyanate stock standard, 17.2 mmol/L (1 mg/L)*. Dissolve 41.8 mg of potassium thiocyanate in 25 mL of de-ionized water.

13. *Thiocyanate working standards, 34.2 and 172.2 µmol/L*. Dilute 100 µL of stock standard to 50 or 10 mL with de-ionized water. Prepare just before use.

Apparatus

1. Conway diffusion cells and covers: polyethylene disk, 60 mm (o.d.); Fisher Scientific no. 08.761/.16 (Bel-Art Products) is suitable.

2. Vacuum grease: Dow Corning "High Vac" grease, or equivalent.

3. Heat source, 40-50 °C: water bath, dry-heat block, or drying oven.

4. Spectrophotometer, visible wavelength range (recording scanning capability desirable, but not required; studies in the Submitters' laboratory were done with a Varian 2290 spectrophotometer, routinely scanning the range 600 to 400 nm).

Specimens

Whole blood is the preferred specimen: the volume used in routine assay is 2 mL, but 1 mL may be used. No additive is necessary, and any of the commonly used anticoagulants are acceptable; specimens retained for several days should be stored at −20 °C.

Gastric specimens are appropriate for confirmation of route of exposure. Urine, serum, or plasma should be used only when whole blood is unavailable to the laboratory; analysis of these specimens should include the direct assay for thiocyanate.

Procedure for Cyanide

1. Label three Conway diffusion cells, A, B, and X.

2. Place a layer of vacuum grease along the entire lip of the cell covers.

3. Pipet 0.5 mL of 0.1 mol/L NaOH solution to the center well of each diffusion cell.

4. Pipet 2 mL of the appropriate blood cyanide standard solution or the sample to the outer ring of the diffusion cells (or to the middle ring in a three-ring cell).

5. Add 0.5 mL of 10 mol/L H_2SO_4 to the outer ring of the diffusion cells, and position the cell covers without delay.

6. Briefly tilt and rotate the diffusion cells to mix the H_2SO_4 with the sample or standard, being careful that none of the sample spills over into the center well.

7. Position the diffusion cells in a uniformly heated environment of 40-50 °C and incubate for 10 min. (Floating the cells on the surface of a water bath at 45 °C was the most frequently used method in the Submitters' laboratory.)

8. Prepare reagent 5 while the diffusion cells are incubating.

9. Remove the diffusion cells to ambient temperature and remove the cell covers.

10. Transfer the contents of the center wells to appropriately labeled tubes (disposable glass 12 × 75 mm tubes are convenient).

11. Place 0.5 mL of 0.1 mol/L NaOH in a tube labeled "blank."

Note: Steps 12-14 are best performed in a fume hood.

12. Add 0.5 mL of 1 mol/L HCl and mix.

13. Add 50 µL of saturated bromine water and mix.

14. Add 200 µL of As_2O_3 solution (reagent 2) and mix.

15. Add 0.8 mL of chromogenic reagent (reagent 5) and mix. Let stand at least 3 min, but proceed to step 16 within 12 min.

16. Measure the peak absorbance of each solution at approximately 490 nm after adjusting the instrument to zero absorbance with water, or record the spectra over the range 400-600 nm (2 nm/s is a satisfactory scanning rate). If using a scanning recording spectrophotometer, the initial and final scans should be overlaid tracings of the high-concentration standard.

17. Construct a standard curve on linear graph paper by plotting the absorbances of the standard solutions (and the blank) vs their concentrations. The plot should yield a straight line. Determine the concentrations of the unknown from this standard curve.

Procedure for Thiocyanate

Note: Perform *only* when whole blood is unavailable.

1. Pipet 0.5 mL of de-ionized water blank, working standard, or sample into appropriately labeled tubes (glass disposable 12 × 75 mm tubes are convenient).

2. Add 4.5 mL of 100 g/L trichloroacetic acid to serum or plasma samples (or 4.5 mL of de-ionized water to urine samples).

3. Vortex-mix for 10 to 15 s and let stand for 5 min.

4. Centrifuge briefly.

5. Transfer 1 mL of supernate into appropriately labeled tubes.

6. Proceed as with the *Procedure for Cyanide*, beginning with step 12.

Results and Discussion

Normal and Abnormal Reference Intervals

Cyanide is normally present in the blood of healthy individuals at concentrations up to 7.7 µmol/L (200 µg/L), the result of vitamin B_{12} metabolism and of environmental factors such as cigarette smoking and ingestion of plants and plant products containing the cyanide glucoside, amygdalin (2, 9, 10). Several investigators (9, 10) have suggested that cyanide concentrations of 19-38 µmol/L (0.50-1.00 mg/L) are associated with mild toxicity, 38-96 µmol/L (1.00-2.50 mg/L) with moderate to severe toxicity, and >96 µmol/L (2.50 mg/L) with fatality unless the patient is promptly subjected to supportive therapy or therapy with specific antidotes. At least two patients (8, 11), including one recently seen in this facility, have completely recovered after prompt specific antidotal treatment, even though cyanide concentrations in the blood exceeded 192 µmol/L (5.0 mg/L). Berlin (12), however, has suggested that because toxicity is related to the intracellular concentration of cyanide, its concentration in blood may be misleading; as a consequence of the tight binding of cyanide to cytochrome oxidase, serious poisoning may occur with modest concentrations in blood, and "certainly any blood level in excess of 20 µg/dL suggests a toxic reaction."

Evaluation of possible cyanide toxicity based on the interpretation of thiocyanate concentrations is considerably less reliable, given the paucity of reliable human data, the relative nonspecificity of some earlier analytical methodologies for thiocyanate, and the chronological patterns of thiocyanate production. Normal plasma concentrations of thiocyanate have been reported as up to 69 µmol/L (4.0 mg/L) for nonsmokers and up to 207 µmol/L (12.0 mg/L) for smokers (12, 13); normal urine concentrations of thiocyanate are reported as up to 69 µmol/L (4.0 mg/L) for nonsmokers and up to 293 µmol/L (17.0 mg/L) for smokers, with >576 µmol/L (30.0 mg/L) being suggestive of acute cyanide toxicity (13, 14). Pontal et al. (15) reported a combined cyanide and thiocyanate urinary excretion of 14.4 mg in 12 h after an acute potassium cyanide ingestion in which blood concentrations of cyanide decreased from an initial 6.0 to 0.80 mg/L 12 h post-ingestion.

Diffusion Conditions

Feldstein (16) discusses in depth the principle and techniques of microdiffusion and describes several of its applications in toxicology, including cyanide analysis. Briefly, if a solution of a volatile substance and a pure solvent are held in separate containers, both of which are in contact with the same atmosphere inside a third sealed container, the volatile solute will pass from the solution into the atmosphere and by gaseous diffusion will be transferred to the surface of the solvent, into which the solute will tend to dissolve. If the solvent is a reagent that converts the volatile solute to a nonvolatile substance and thereby reduces its vapor pressure almost to zero, no equilibrium is reached, so that eventually all of the volatile solute diffuses into the reagent and remains there. Addition of acid to a solution of cyanide ions produces volatile hydrogen cyanide, which then diffuses and eventually dissolves in dilute alkali solution, where hydrogen cyanide is converted to the nonvolatile alkali cyanide salt.

Conway diffusion cells are available in different sizes and in at least two different designs. As Feldstein states (16), "The diffusion characteristics for each of these units (diffusion cells) must be investigated individually, and the effects of time, temperature and volume on the completeness of diffusion should be determined for each apparatus"; this should be borne in mind while reviewing the described procedure. The diffusion cells used in the Submitters' laboratory are the modified three-ring cells, 6 cm in diameter. The center well contains the dilute alkali to "fix" the cyanide ions as sodium salts, the middle ring contains the specimen and the "liberating" acid, and the outer ring is sealed with the sealant grease and is fastened with the cover. In the development of the described procedure, the volume and chemical nature of the acid and the concentration of the sodium hydroxide solution were used as described by Pettigrew and Fell (4) without further evaluation; the volume of sodium hydroxide solution, though different from what they used, was determined by the type and size of Conway diffusion cell available and hence was not evaluated. Similarly, we did not evaluate techniques of maintaining continuous motion of the fluid surfaces through use of shakers or rotators.

In the initial studies, the Submitters used 1.8 mol/L sulfuric acid, the concentration used by Pettigrew and Fell to convert cyanide ion to hydrogen cyanide. The later studies were performed with 10 mol/L sulfuric acid, McAnalley et al. (17) having reported that sulfuric acid concentrations of 1 to 10 mol/L were satisfactory, with the rate of release increasing with the concentration of the acid. Our data indicated that, for a 10-min diffusion at 45 °C, sensitivity increased approximately 32% as the acid concentration increased from 1.0 to 4.0 mol/L; the sensitivity increased less as the concentration was further increased up to 10 mol/L.

Diffusion proceeds more rapidly at higher temperatures, so that higher concentrations of cyanide are captured in the sodium hydroxide solution after shorter periods of diffusion. Three types of heat sources generally present in analytical toxicology laboratories were evaluated: diffusion cells were placed within a drying oven, on the surface of dry-heat blocks, or floated in a water bath. Results by each method were comparable, as long as the standards and specimen were treated the same. The temperatures we evaluated ranged from a low ambient temperature through higher temperatures that would be expected to be easily available at any time in a toxicology laboratory—that is, a drying oven would be on hand to expedite presumptive colorimetric tests or develop ninhydrin-sprayed chromatographic plates, a water bath would be available to enhance sensitivity of head-space gas-chromatographic analysis for alcohols, and dry-heat blocks would be used to expedite evaporation of solvent extracts. The rate of diffusion increased with temperature over the range studied, but precision was poorer at temperatures greater than 55 °C (Table 1). We selected 45 °C as a

Table 1. Influence of Temperature on Extent of Diffusion

Submitters' data		Evaluators' data[b]		
Temp, °C	% total diffusion, mean ± SD[a]	Temp, °C	Absorbance	Recovery, %
22	37.6 ± 0.1	25	1.476 ± 0.050	28 ± 1.2
35	42.5 ± 1.4	35	1.721 ± 0.050	31 ± 1.2
45	49.3 ± 1.0	45	1.820 ± 0.090	37 ± 2.3
55	51.7 ± 4.4	55	2.495 ± 0.190	49 ± 3.2
65	59.3 ± 2.6	65	3.140 ± 0.180	53 ± 3.1

[a] After 20-min diffusion of aqueous cyanide standard, 10.4 µg/L, in a diffusion cell floated on a water bath.
[b] Results are mean ± SD (n = 5) for 2 mL of whole blood containing cyanide at 38.5 µmol/L, diffused 10 min.

Table 2. Effect of Temperature and Duration of Diffusion

Submitters: relative absorbance[a]			Evaluators: % recovery[b]					
	Diffusion time, min			Diffusion time, min				
Temp, °C	10	20	Temp, °	2	4	8	12	16
22	1.0	1.6	25	7	14	23	30	39
45	1.9	2.1	45	13	21	31	47	51

[a] Mean ratio of absorbance measured to that at 22 °C after 10 min of diffusion (n = 5 each).
[b] Percent of cyanide recovered from whole blood containing 38.5 µmol of cyanide per liter (average of duplicate determinations).

suitable temperature for routine analyses, the sensitivity at this temperature being about twice that achieved at ambient temperature with no appreciable loss of precision. This temperature was also convenient, because we continually maintain a water bath at this temperature in our laboratory for support of other tests.

The quantity of cyanide transferred from the specimen to the sodium hydroxide solution is a function of the duration of the diffusion; however, the increased transfer with extended time is less pronounced as the temperature increases because more of the cyanide diffuses sooner (Table 2). A 10-min diffusion at 45 °C is suggested for emergency analysis of blood cyanide, even though only about one-fourth of the cyanide will be recovered in the sodium hydroxide solution under these conditions. Nonetheless, this provides adequate sensitivity and precision and, whereas sensitivity is increased more than threefold by extending the diffusion from 5 to 10 min, a further extension to 15 min increased sensitivity by only about 50%.

Rinsing the center well with 0.5 mL of de-ionized water after sodium hydroxide solution had been transferred did not significantly enhance precision, and the small increase in the quantity of sodium cyanide transferred was more than offset by the additional dilution, which resulted in a lower absorbance. Consequently, the recommended routine technique is a single transfer of sample with a glass Pasteur pipet.

Because blood cyanide is predominantly bound intracellularly within erythrocytes (2), we examined the influence of the surfactant octoxynol (Triton X-100) upon the diffusion of cyanide from whole blood. Before analysis, whole blood containing 2.00 mg of cyanide per liter was vortex-mixed for 2 min with 50 mL/L aqueous Triton X-100 at ratios of blood to surfactant solution ranging from 1:0.05 to 1:2. More cyanide was recovered from samples mixed with a 1:1 or greater ratio of blood to surfactant volumes, but there was no improvement in precision, and the measured absorbance decreased as a consequence of the dilution.

Chromogenic Reaction

Bromine reagent (reagent 1). Both commercially available saturated bromine water and saturated aqueous solution prepared from and stored in contact with reagent-grade bromine are satisfactory. Bromine concentration may be expected to decrease with time unless the solution is stored in contact with excess bromine, or the container is always securely sealed. Under the conditions described, there was no significant reduction in sensitivity or precision over the range of 30 to 100% saturation, and sensitivity decreased by only 8% at 10% saturation; consequently, the problems generally associated with the use of saturated solutions are minimized, unless solutions are stored for prolonged periods in the absence of excess bromine. On the other hand, a potential problem with solutions stored in contact with excess bromine is that, should the pipet tip be inserted into the liquid bromine or rubbed against the sides of the container, a great excess of bromine may be delivered into the tube, in which case the sample immediately turns intensely purple when the chromogenic reagent is added.

Bromination. Pettigrew and Fell (4) used two drops of bromine solution and three drops of arsenous oxide solution, then briefly evaporated the sample at reduced pressure and increased temperature to eliminate any excess bromine. In the method we report here, precision and sensitivity were significantly improved by using *measured* quantities of the bromine and arsenous oxide reagent (50 and 200 µL, respectively) and eliminating the evaporation step. Extending the time between addition of the hydrochloric acid, bromine solution, arsenous oxide solution, and chromogenic reagent from 30 s to 10 min did not significantly affect precision or sensitivity.

Color development and measurement. Although Pettigrew and Fell used 1.8 mL of chromogenic reagent (reagent 5), we noted an enhanced sensitivity with no change in precision as the volume of reagent was decreased to about 0.8 mL, thus decreasing the dilution of the resulting colored product; both precision and sensitivity diminished when the volume of chromogenic reagent was less than 0.6 mL (Table 3).

To minimize variations in measured absorbance with time, Pettigrew and Fell recommended measuring at the isosbestic point (the common intercept of spectra recorded at different times after the chromogenic reaction) for this

Table 3. Effect of Different Volumes of Chromogenic Reagent

Reagent vol, mL	Absorbance[a]		CV, %
	Mean	SD	
1.8	0.672	0.006	0.9
1.5	0.820	0.004	0.4
1.2	0.847	0.004	0.5
1.0	0.946	0.008	0.8
0.8	1.000	0.001	0.1
0.6	0.982	0.004	0.4
0.4	0.830	0.025	3.0
0.2	0.153	0.004	2.6

[a] Absorbance at 490 nm, presented as ratio of absorbance obtained with 0.8 mL of reagent (n = 5 each).

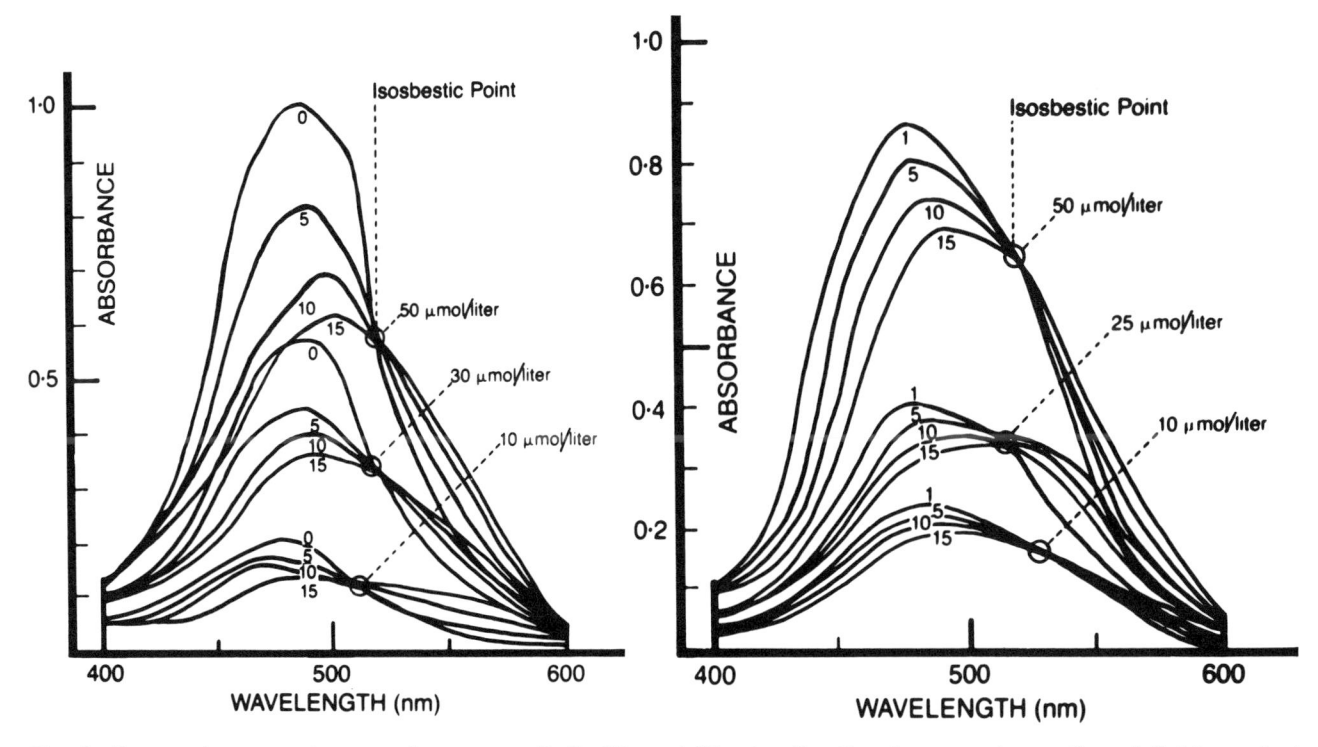

Fig. 1. Repeated spectrophotometric scans at 0, 5, 10, and 15 min after the chromogenic reaction of *(left)* standard solutions of potassium thiocyanate subjected to the colorimetric procedure of Pettigrew and Fell *(4)*, and *(right)* standard solutions of potassium cyanide subjected to the modified colorimetric procedure described here

reaction (~ 520 nm), instead of at the point of maximum absorbance (~ 490 nm) (Figure 1, left); they also noted the necessity to redetermine the isosbestic point for each new batch of reagents.

Measurement of absorbance is slightly less time-dependent under the conditions described here (Figure 1, right). Pettigrew and Fell noted that for a 50 μmol/L solution of thiocyanate, absorbance decreased by about 25% and the absorbance peak shifted by 12 nm from 5 to 15 min after addition of chromogenic reagent; for a 50 μmol/L solution of cyanide, we observed a 12% decrease in absorbance and a 9-nm shift over the same period. Generally, if peak absorbances are measured within 7 ± 4 min of the start of the chromogenic reaction, the coefficient of variation (CV) for replicate determinations will be approximately 3%.

Pettigrew and Fell also noted that the apparent isosbestic point is a function of concentration, shifting for one reagent batch from 512 nm for a 10 μmol/L solution of cyanide to 508 nm for a 50 μmol/L solution. They recommended that readings be taken within 10 min at a wavelength known to be the isosbestic point for this reaction. However, we find that, if a manual nonrecording spectrophotometer is used, all measurements should be made at the wavelength of maximum absorbance for the highest concentration standard, all at the same interval (± 1 min) after the reaction is initiated. This is easily done by appropriately spacing the addition of the chromogenic reagent to the blank, standards, and sample(s). For use with the recording spectrophotometer, we recommend that the initial and final measurements be an overlay of the high-concentration standard, with the blank, low-concentration standard, and specimen(s) measured in between. This allows one to determine the isosbestic point, and hence provides greater precision, at the expense of only the time required for one additional scan.

General Comments

The described method allows the rapid and simple determination of blood cyanide, and requires no apparatus or instrumentation that is not usually present in even the smallest toxicology laboratory. The microdiffusion technique is considerably less tedious than methods involving steam distillation or aeration with gas-washing tubes *(18)*, and the colorimetric detection method is more sensitive than direct measurement with a cyanide ion-selective electrode *(18)*.

Most methods for quantifying blood cyanide by microdiffusion have relied on quantification of nondiffused aqueous standards. This approach is satisfactory when the diffusion is allowed to proceed from 2 to 4 h to achieve essentially complete recovery of the cyanide *(16,17)*, but extended diffusion times generally translate into actual turnaround times of at least 3 to 5 h in the clinical setting when set-up and calibration are included. Actual complete turnaround time may be reduced to about 40 min by using a much shorter diffusion time. Turnaround time also depends on practical laboratory management, which includes periodically checking that the necessary reagents and apparatus are appropriately grouped and that reagents of limited stability are available when required (reagents 3 and 4 of this procedure should be prepared at least quarterly).

However, the incomplete cyanide recovery, resulting from the shorter diffusion time, requires the use of standards that have been similarly diffused. Further, at the shorter diffusion time proposed for emergency toxicology analysis, the slower release of hydrogen cyanide from blood than from water means that quantification should be based on similarly diffused standards of cyanide in blood. McAnalley et al. *(17)* argued against the use of blood cyanide standards, "because normal blood contains a significant and variable amount of cyanide ion"; however, the cyanide content they reported from the analysis of 100 random blood specimens ranged from approximately 1.9 to 3.1 µmol/L, in agreement with Ballantyne's (19) report of a mean normal blood cyanide concentration of 1.9 µmol/L. Studies in the Submitters' laboratory suggest a mean normal blood cyanide concentration of 3.0 µmol/L, 3.7 µmol/L being the highest concentration detected in an unselected specimen. These concentrations do not seem sufficient to preclude the use of blood standards for emergency toxicology assays, given that the lowest blood cyanide concentrations generally associated with mild and moderate to severe toxicity are 19 and 39 µmol/L, respectively.

The described method is capable of detecting blood cyanide at 2 µmol/L and the standard curve is linear over the range of 10 to 160 µmol/L (Table 4). The final colored solutions may be diluted with de-ionized water as much as fourfold if the absorbance of a sample exceeds the spectrophotometric range of the instrument used.

Table 4. Spectrophotometric Response to Cyanide Concentrations Added to Blood

Cyanide concentration, µmol/L (mg/L)	Absorbance at 490 nm[a]
154 (4.0)	3.812 ± 0.090
77 (2.0)	1.805 ± 0.147
38.5 (1.0)	0.953 ± 0.029
19.2 (0.5)	0.543 ± 0.015
9.6 (0.25)	0.325 ± 0.006
0	0.100 ± 0.020

[a] Mean ± SD (n = 5).

Evaluators' Notes

The Submitters, using a 60-mm diffusion cell, reported a mean recovery of 25% for a 10-min diffusion at 45 °C for 2 mL of whole blood to which 38.5 µmol of cyanide had been added per tube. The Evaluators recovered 20% of the added cyanide with similar cells at the same concentration and conditions, but recovered 37% with a 83-mm-diameter diffusion cell, because of the greater surface area. The data submitted by the Evaluators for Tables 1, 2, and 5 were obtained with the larger diffusion cells. Moreover, although the Submitters reported that precision diminished as the diffusion temperature was increased above 45 °C, the Evaluators did not observe poorer precision through 65 °C. The Evaluators' data concur with the Submitters' conclusions concerning limits of detection and linearity, and of precision. However, the Evaluators did not find that acceptable linearity could be achieved by diluting the final colored solution if absorbance exceeded the instrument's range; rather, they recommend that in the event of excessive absorbance, a preliminary report should state that the concentration of blood cyanide exceeds a specified value, and that the analysis be repeated with a smaller specimen volume or

Table 5. Spectrophotometric Response to Different Cyanide Concentrations

Cyanide concn, µmol/L	Absorbance at 490 nm, mean ± SD (and CV, %)	% recovery
1.0	0.079 ± 0.010 (8.6)	49
1.9	0.112 ± 0.004 (2.2)	45
3.9	0.175 ± 0.004 (1.8)	45
7.7	0.309 ± 0.004 (1.4)	44
19.2	0.640 ± 0.010 (1.5)	44
38.5	1.208 ± 0.060 (4.9)	37
154	2.455 ± 0.140 (2.9)	37

Evaluators' data: diffusion time, 10 min at 45 °C. n = 5 each.

by diluting the sodium hydroxide solution of diffused cyanide before the chromogenic reaction.

References

1. Cohen L. Cyanide. *Poison Dig* **2**(2), 1-5 (1983).
2. Graham DL, Laman D, Theodore J, Robin ED. Acute cyanide poisoning complicated by lactic acidosis and pulmonary edema. *Arch Intern Med* **137**, 1051-1055 (1977).
3. Vogel SN, Sultan TR, Ten Eyck RP. Cyanide poisoning. *Clin Toxicol* **18**, 367-383 (1981).
4. Pettigrew AR, Fell GS. Simplified colorimetric determination of thiocyaniate in biologic fluids, and its application to investigation of toxic amblyopias. *Clin Chem* **18**, 996-1000 (1972).
5. Bark LS, Higson HG. A review of methods available for the detection and determination of small amounts of cyanide. *Analyst (London)* **88**, 751 (1963).
6. König WJ. Verfahren zur Darstellung neuer stickstoffhaltiger Farbstoffe. *Angew Chem* **11**, 115 (1905).
7. Pettigrew AR, Fell GS. Microdiffusion method for estimation of cyanide in whole blood and its application to the study of conversion of cyanide to thiocyanate. *Clin Chem* **19**, 466-471 (1973).
8. Friauf B, Poirot C. Kit helps treat poisoning. *Fort Worth Star Telegram*, March 11, 1983.
9. Bauman J. Cyanide. In *Poison Information Bulletin*, National Poison Center Network, Pittsburgh, PA, 1983.
10. Stewart R. Cyanide poisoning. *Clin Toxicol* **7**, 561-564 (1974).
11. Bain JT, Knowles EL. Successful treatment of cyanide poisoning. *Br Med J* **ii**, 763 (1967).
12. Berlin C. Cyanide poisoning—a challenge. *Arch Intern Med* **137**, 993-994 (1977).
13. Basalt RC. *Analytical Procedures for Therapeutic Drug Monitoring and Emergency Toxicology*, Biomedical Publications, Davis, CA, 1980, pp 275-277.
14. *The Bioscience Handbook of Clinical and Industrial Toxicology*, Bioscience Laboratories, Van Nuys, CA, 1979, p 85.
15. Pontal PG, Bismuth C, Garnier R, Pronczuk de Garbino J. Therapeutic attitude in cyanide poisoning: Retrospective study of 24 non-lethal cases. *Vet Hum Toxicol* **24** (suppl), 90-93 (1982).
16. Feldstein M. Microdiffusion analysis as applied to toxicology. In *Toxicology*, I, CP Stewart, A Stolman, Eds., Academic Press, New York, NY, 1960, pp 639-659.
17. McAnalley BH, Lowry WR, Oliver RD, Garriott JC. Determination of inorganic sulfide and cyanide in blood using specific ion electrodes: Application to the investigation of hydrogen sulfide and cyanide poisoning. *J Anal Toxicol* **3**, 111 (1979).
18. Egekeze JO, Oehme FW. Direct potentiometric methods for the determination of cyanide in biological materials. *J Anal Toxicol* **3**, 119 (1979).
19. Ballantyne B. Postmortem rate of transformation of cyanide. *Forensic Sci* **3**, 71 (1974).

Ethanol in Biological Fluids by Enzymic Analysis

Submitters: Richard H. Gadsden, Sr., and E. Howard Taylor, *Department of Laboratory Medicine, Medical University of South Carolina, Charleston, SC 29425*

Evaluators: Steven J. Steindel, *Piedmont Hospital, Atlanta, GA 30309*
Francis A. Ragan, Jr., and Karl M. Doetsch, *L.S.U. Medical Center, Department of Pathology, New Orleans, LA 70112*

Introduction

The enzymic method for determining the ethanol (EtOH) content in fluids is especially useful when only low concentrations of EtOH are present.[1] The use of alcohol dehydrogenase (ADH; alcohol:NAD$^+$ oxidoreductase, EC 1.1.1.1) for this is relatively specific for EtOH (*1,2*), and several published methods utilizing this principle are quite suitable for clinical purposes (*3-5*).

The principle here is based on the method of Bucher and Redetzki (*3*), in which EtOH is oxidized by nicotine adenine dinucleotide (NAD$^+$) in the presence of ADH with the resulting formation of acetaldehyde and NADH:

$$CH_3CH_2OH + NAD^+ \longleftrightarrow CH_3CHO + NADH + H^+$$

A high ratio of enzyme/coenzyme to substrate is maintained so that equilibrium is reached relatively quickly.

Bucher and Redetzki (*3*) recommended including semicarbazide to drive the reaction to the right by converting the acetaldehyde to its respective hydrozone. In the method set forth here we use tris(hydroxymethyl)-aminomethane (Tris) as a "trapping" agent (*6*) for the acetaldehyde, and as the buffer.

The conversion of EtOH to acetaldehyde proceeds rapidly and the formation of NADH is monitored spectrophotometrically at 340 nm.

The method may be used to measure EtOH in serum, plasma, whole blood, vitreous fluid, and urine. Grossly hemolyzed serum or plasma and whole blood require pretreatment with trichloroacetic acid (TCA) before analysis of the resulting supernate. We have also used this method for homogenized solid-tissue specimens after treatment with TCA.

Materials and Methods

Reagents

ADH from yeast (Sigma Chemical Co., St. Louis, MO 63178; cat. no. A7011, 75 kU per vial). Dissolve contents of the vial in 100 mL of distilled water (final concentration, 750 U/mL). Stored in convenient small volumes (1-2 mL), sealed with Parafilm, and kept frozen (-20 to -70 °C), these are stable for about three months.

NAD$^+$ (coenzyme I; M_r 694.48). Obtained from Sigma Chemical Co., cat. no. N0632, Grade VII, sodium salt, 5 g per vial (contains approximately 4.5 g of NAD$^+$). Dissolve in 100 mL of distilled water (final concentration, about 70 mmol/mL). Aliquot, and store frozen like ADH. Stable for about three months.

Evaluator S.J.S. found the stability of the reagents ADH and NAD$^+$ to be poor at room and refrigerator temperature. He did not evaluate stability at -20 to -70 °C.

ADH/NAD$^+$ working solution. Thaw an aliquot of the ADH and NAD$^+$ solutions and mix together in equal volumes. (The manual method requires 0.2 mL of the ADH/NAD$^+$ solution per determination.) Final concentrations per reaction mixture: about 75 U of ADH and about 7 mol of NAD$^+$.

Tris buffer, 0.5 mol/L, pH 8.8 ± 0.1. Dissolve 60.5 g of Tris (Fisher Scientific Co., Pittsburgh, PA 15238; "THAM," cat. no. 5-395, ACS grade) in about 750 mL of distilled water; adjust the pH to 8.9 ± 0.1 with HCl (1 mol/L). Dilute to 1 L with distilled water. The reagent is stable under refrigeration; keep a small volume (50-100 mL) at room temperature for ready use.

EtOH stock standard. Do all pipeting and weighing at room temperature. Pre-weigh a 50-mL GS volumetric flask containing about 25 mL of distilled water (this prevents absorption of atmospheric water when absolute EtOH is added to the flask). Add 4 mL of absolute EtOH (reagent quality; AAPER Alcohol and Chemical Co., Shelbyville, KY 40065) and reweigh. Calculate the weight of the EtOH by the difference in weights. Dilute to 50 mL with distilled water. This stock standard is stable when refrigerated and protected against evaporation. Bring an appropriate aliquot to room temperature before preparing working standards. (See section on *Quality Control* for additional sources of primary EtOH standards.)

EtOH working standards. Pipet 5, 2.5, 2, and 1 mL of the EtOH stock standard into individual 100-mL GS volumetric flasks and add distilled water to volume. Mix well by inversion. Protect against evaporation. Standards are stable under refrigeration.

Example: At a room temperature of 20 °C the 4 mL of EtOH (density = 0.78945 g/mL) would weigh 3.1578 g (*7*). The concentrations of the working standards would thus be 3158, 1580, 1263, and 632 mg/L, respectively.

Quality Control

Whole-blood controls are available from Fisher Scientific, Diagnostics Div., Orangeburg, NY 10962, and serum controls from Ortho Diagnostics Systems, Inc., Raritan,

---

[1] Nonstandard abbreviations: EtOH, ethanol; ADH, alcohol dehydrogenase; TCA, trichloroacetic acid.

NJ 08869, and contain EtOH only. Certified aqueous primary EtOH is available from the National Bureau of Standards, Washington, DC 20234, or from the American College of Pathologists, 7400 N. Skokie Blvd., Skokie, IL 60077. A certified and working (secondary) aqueous EtOH standard is available from MCB Manufacturing Chemists, Inc., Gibbstown, NJ 08027. An appropriate quality-control specimen should be included in each analytical run.

Procedure

Manual (macro) method for serum or plasma. Reagents should be at room temperature. Pipet into 5- to 7-mL test tubes 2.8 mL of Tris buffer and 0.2 mL of ADH/NAD$^+$. For the blank add 10 µL of distilled water and to the other tubes add 10 µL of standards or serum (or plasma), respectively. Cover each with Parafilm and mix by inversion. After incubating the tubes at 30-37 °C for 15 min, transfer their contents to cuvettes. Set the blank at zero absorbance at 340 nm, then measure the absorbance of the standards and samples. Plot the absorbance of the standards vs concentration, then determine the concentration of EtOH in the samples from the graph. The standard curve is linear from 0 to 3250 mg of EtOH per liter. Samples with EtOH exceeding 3000 mg/L should be diluted threefold and redetermined; multiply the result by three (the dilution factor) to obtain final result.

Evaluator F.A.R. suggested preparing a mixture of the Tris buffer and ADH/NAD$^+$ at a ratio of 30:2 and pipeting 3.0 mL of this reagent for each sample. This convenient approach maintained the linearity, intercept, and slope of the standard curve.

Note: If the specimen to be analyzed is whole blood or is grossly hemolyzed, prepare a protein-free supernate by treating 1 mL of blood with 2 mL of TCA (60 g/L). Cover the sample with Parafilm and mix well for 5 min. Centrifuge (5 min, 3000 × g) and use 10 µL of the clear supernate as the sample. Multiply the analytical result by the dilution factor of 3. (This also applies to the micro method.)

Micro method for serum or plasma (semiautomated, centrifugal analyzer: GEMSAEC, Electro-Nucleonics, Inc., Fairfield, NJ 07006). Dilute standard(s) and sample 10-fold with distilled water. To test tubes containing 280 µL of Tris buffer + 20 µL of ADH/NAD$^+$ solution add 10 µL of distilled water (blank), 10 µL of diluted standard, or 10 µL of diluted sample. Allow the reaction to proceed for 15 min at 30-37 °C, then determine the concentration of EtOH in the unknowns as in the manual (macro) method.

Results and Discussion

The working standards were analyzed in quadruplicate by the manual (macro) method in development of a standard curve (Figure 1). This reaction is linear and reproducible from 0 to 3158 mg/L of EtOH. Similar results are obtained for pooled serum samples and the semiautomated (micro) method.

Evaluator F.A.R. found the standard curve to be linear to 3158 mg of EtOH. The paired-value statistics were: a = 0.007; b = 0.9145; $S_{y/x}$ = 0.01; r = 0.9933; bias = 0.00; SD = 0.01.

To determine the optimum reaction temperature and time, we analyzed an EtOH standard of 3000 mg/L by the manual (macro) method, letting the reaction proceed for 30 min and reading absorbance, at the frequency shown in Figure 2 (the plot has been cropped to 15 min for illustration). The reaction was carried out at room temperature (22 °C), 30, and 37 °C. The reaction at room temperature reaches equilibrium at about 25 min. At 30 and 37 °C the reaction attains equilibrium in 10 min. The latter temperatures (range) are recommended for the method for convenience and reproducibility.

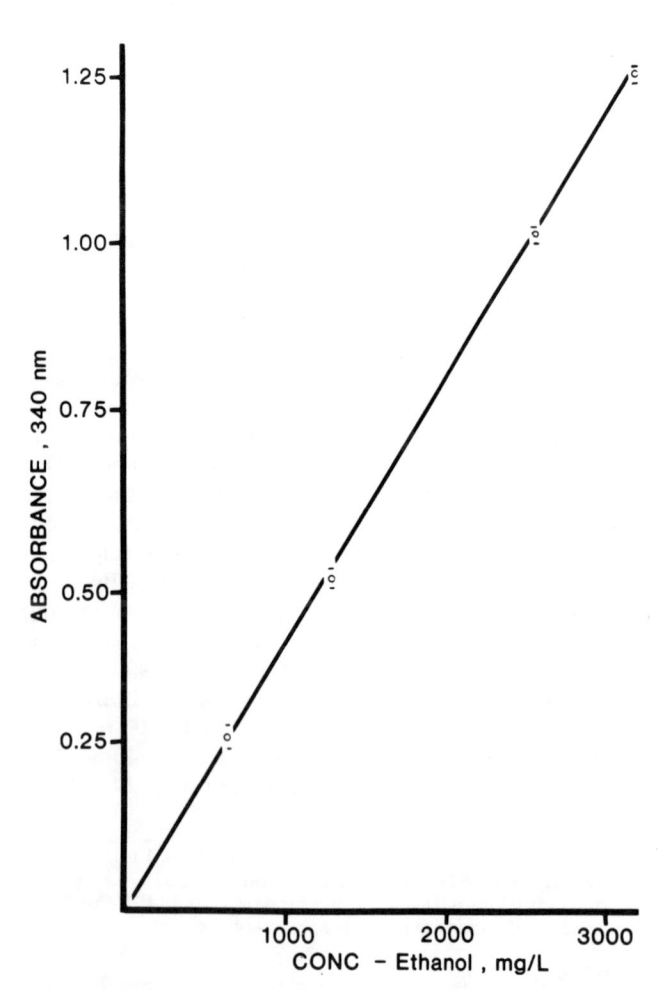

Fig. 1. Standard curve for enzymic analysis of ethanol
Ethanol concentrations as stated in Table 1; results (o) are the means of replicate analyses (n = 5). Measurements were made after 15 min at 37 °C

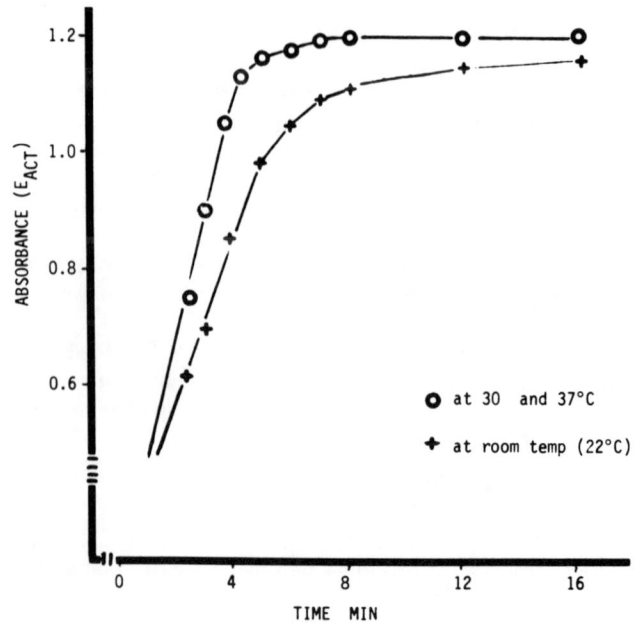

Fig. 2. ADH activity vs time and temperature
Zero-order kinetics are attained at 30-37 °C. Ethanol, 3000 mg/L

Interference. We investigated some volatile solvents commonly encountered in intoxicated patients as possible interferents with this method. Isopropanol at 950 mg/L gave an apparent EtOH content of 65 mg/L; methanol at 1000 mg/L, 31 mg/L; ethylene glycol at 1100 mg/L, 40 mg/L; acetone at 1200 mg/L, 0 mg/L. These interferences should not be considered clinically significant.

Precision and recovery. Human pooled serum, found to be EtOH-free by gas chromatography, was used to prepare protein-based EtOH solutions, as was described above for aqueous working standards of EtOH. These were analyzed in replicate by the described method. The target values were verified by gas chromatography. Table 1 summarizes these data in terms of precision and recovery.

Table 1. Determination of EtOH in Serum-Based Samples[a]

EtOH, mg/L

Target value	Mean	SD	Range (and % recovery)	CV, %
496	495	25.9	470-519 (94.9-104.8)	5.2
994	994	25.1	965-1027 (97.1-103.3)	2.5
1980	1980	49.6	1908-2086 (96.3-105.4)	2.5
2973	2975	88.9	2766-3082 (93.0-103.6)	3.0

[a] Replicate samples assayed in duplicate on 18 different days (n = 36).

Evaluator S.J.S. evaluated the method's accuracy by comparing it with that of the Du Pont *aca* ALC/ADH method. The mean for patients' samples analyzed with the *aca* was 1611 mg/L; that by the Selected Method was 1515 mg/L (n = 18), significantly different (Student's *t*-test) at $p = 0.004$. A linear regression study of the data gave a slope of 0.925, an intercept of 26 mg/L, $r = 0.992$, and SEM = 104 mg/L. S.J.S. states that the major difference between the methods can be directly traced to calibration differences.

Note: The Selected Method and the gas-chromatographic head-space method were calibrated with the working standards described. Analysis of patients' plasma (n = 100) by the Selected Method (x) and head-space method (y) gave linear regression statistics of: slope = 0.9970, intercept = -0.089, $r = 0.9970$, mean $x = 157.6$ (SD 59.3), mean $y = 159.3$ (SD 60.2).

Comments:

1. Use a spectrophotometer with a 10-nm band-pass and cuvettes with a 1-cm light path.
2. Monitor the absorbance of the blank (Tris + ADH/NAD$^+$) vs Tris buffer. When the blank absorbance exceeds 0.100, prepare fresh NAD$^+$ solution and ADH/NAD$^+$ reagent.
3. The total standard curve need not be repeated in each run as long as the ADH/NAD$^+$ reagent maintains its quality. After the initial standardization, include the approximate 1000 and 3000 mg/L standards in subsequent analytical runs.
4. Run all standards in duplicate within each run. The approximate 1000 mg/L standard should agree within ±5% and the 3000 mg/L standard within ±3%.
5. Single-assay vials containing NAD$^+$ (1.8 mol) and ADH (150 U) are available from Sigma Chemical Co. (NAD-ADH single assay vial, stock no. 330-1) and are stable for at least one year when kept refrigerated. Dissolve the contents of each vial in 3 mL of Tris buffer before adding standard or sample. Multi-assay vials are also available from Sigma Chemical Co. (stock no. 332-5); Calbiochem, Summerville, NJ 08876 ("Alcohol Stat-Pak", cat. no. 869-219) and Boehringer-Mannheim Diagnostics, Indianapolis, IN 46250 (Alcohol, cat. no. 123960) have reagents available in kit form. DuPont Clinical Systems Div., Wilmington, DE 19898, has developed a rapid alcohol (ALC) method for the *aca* that is useful for "stat" determinations. We have found that results by these methods correlate well with those by this Selected Method.

References

1. Barron ESG, Levine S. Oxidation of alcohols by yeast alcohol dehydrogenase and by living cells. *Arch Biochem Biophys* 41, 175-187 (1952).
2. Jones D, Gerber LP, Drell W. A rapid enzymatic method for estimating ethanol in body fluids. *Clin Chem* 16, 402-407 (1970).
3. Bucher T, Redetzki H. Eine spezifische photometriche Bestimmung von Äthylalkohol auf fermatativen Wege. *Klin Wochenschr* 29, 615-617 (1951).
4. Bonnichsen RK, Theorell H. An enzymatic method for the micro determination of ethanol. *Scand J Clin Lab Invest* 3, 58-62 (1951).
5. Brink NG, Bonnichsen RK, Theorell H. A modified method for the enzymatic microdetermination of ethanol. *Acta Pharmacol Toxicol* 10, 223-226 (1954).
6. *Merck Index*, 9th ed., Merck and Co., Inc., Rahway, NJ, 1976, p 1253.
7. *Handbook of Chemistry and Physics*, 62nd ed., CRC Press, Inc., Boca Raton, FL, 1981-1982, p F-3 (table).

Ethchlorvynol by Spectrophotometry

Submitter: Christopher S. Frings, *Medical Laboratory Associates, Birmingham, AL 35256*

Evaluators: Cecelia H. Queen, *Duckworth Pathology Group, Memphis, TN 38104*

C. Ray Ratliff, *Bio-Analytic Laboratories, Inc., Palm City, FL 33490*

Introduction

Ethchlorvynol (1-chloro-3-ethyl-1-penten-4-yl-3-ol, "Placidyl®"; Abbott Laboratories, North Chicago, IL 60644) is a nonbarbiturate hypnotic.

Algeri et al. (1) reported a colorimetric method for determining ethchlorvynol, based on the reaction of the allyl group with phloroglucinol in concentrated hydrochloric acid. The procedure of Wallace et al. (2) is based on the formation of a carbonyl derivative of the drug by reaction of its vinyl chloride group in acid solution. Robinson (3) described a gas-chromatographic method for determining ethchlorvynol in serum and urine.

Weinberg and Dal Cortivo (4) and Frings and Cohen (5) described methods based on the formation of a pink reaction product of ethchlorvynol with diphenylamine, sulfuric acid, and acetic acid. The latter method has been widely used for several years and was published in 1972 in *Standard Methods of Clinical Chemistry* (6).

Principle

The method of Frings and Cohen (5,6) for determining ethchlorvynol in serum, gastric contents, and urine depends on the formation of a colored product when diphenylamine, sulfuric acid, and acetic acid are added to an ethchlorvynol-containing sample from which protein has been precipitated by trichloroacetic acid. The absorbance of this product at 510 nm is proportional to the ethchlorvynol concentration.

Materials and Methods

Reagents

1. *Trichloroacetic acid (TCA):* Dissolve 100 g of TCA in de-ionized water and dilute to 1 L with de-ionized water. This solution is stable for six months when stored in a brown glass bottle at 2-6 °C.

2. *Ethchlorvynol color reagent:* Add 50 mL of concentrated sulfuric acid containing 1.0 g of diphenylamine to 100 mL of aqueous acetic acid (equal volumes of water and acetic acid). This solution is stable for one year when stored in a brown glass bottle at room temperature.

3. *Ethchlorvynol stock standard, 1.00 g/L:* Dilute 100.0 mg of ethchlorvynol to 100 mL with absolute ethanol in a volumetric flask. This solution is stable for two months when stored in a tightly capped brown glass bottle at 2-6 °C.

4. *Ethchlorvynol working standard, 20 mg/L:* Dilute 2.0 mL of stock standard to 100 mL with de-ionized water in a volumetric flask. This solution is stable for one month when stored in a brown glass bottle at 2-6 °C.

Apparatus

1. A 10-nm or lower band-pass spectrometer or spectrophotometer.
2. Water bath, 37 ± 2 °C.

Collection and Handling of Specimens

Serum is the preferred sample for quantitative analysis. Urine, gastric contents, serum, and plasma are all suitable for qualitative analysis. Samples are stable for several days when stored at 2-6 °C and for months when stored frozen.

Quantitative Procedure for Serum Samples

1. To each of four 16 × 100 mm tubes add 4.5 mL of TCA solution.
2. To the first tube (blank) add 0.50 mL of water.
3. To the second tube (standard) add 0.50 mL of 20 mg/L working standard.
4. To the third tube (control) add 0.50 mL of control.
5. To the fourth tube (unknown) add 0.50 mL of serum or urine.
6. Vortex-mix the contents of each tube for at least 30 s.
7. Centrifuge for 10 min at 750 × g.
8. To appropriately labeled 16 × 150 mm tubes add 2.0 mL of protein-free filtrate from blank, standard, control, and unknown.
9. Add 3.0 mL of color reagent to each tube and vortex-mix.
10. Incubate all tubes at 37 (±2) °C for 30 min.
11. Cool for 5 min at room temperature.
12. Within an additional 5 min measure the absorbance (A) of the standard and unknown at 510 nm against the blank.
13. Calculate the concentration of ethchlorvynol as follows:

$$\frac{A\ unknown}{A\ standard} \times 20 = \text{concentration, mg/L}$$

Because ethchlorvynol is a synthetic compound, its normal concentration in humans is zero. A serum concentration of ethchlorvynol <1 mg/L obtained by this method should be reported as none detected.

Qualitative Screening Procedure (Urine or Gastric Contents)

This short method is to be used only for the qualitative detection of ethchlorvynol in urine or gastric contents and is not suitable for serum. Use the quantitative procedure (above) when the concentration of ethchlorvynol in serum is requested.

1. Add 0.2 mL of urine control to a tube (control).
2. Add 0.2 mL of urine or gastric contents to a second tube (unknown).
3. Add 1.8 mL of the TCA solution to each tube and vortex-mix.
4. Add 2.0 mL of color reagent to each tube and mix well.
5. Incubate all tubes at 37 (±2) °C for 15 min.

A pink color is positive for ethchlorvynol. Report results as either positive or none detected.

Results and Discussion

Expected values. In adults who ingested single 1-g doses of ethchlorvynol, the concentration in blood reached a maximum of 14 mg/L within 1 to 1.5 h; thereafter, the concentration gradually decreased to "zero" (none detected) 4 h after ingestion (2). Patients have recovered after ingesting 10 to 25 g of ethchlorvynol, but some persons have died with a blood concentration of about 140 mg/L.

Table 1. Analytical Recovery of Ethchlorvynol from Serum and Urine[a]

Ethchlorvynol, mg/L		
Added	Recovered	Recovery, %
Serum		
5	5	100
5	5	100
10	10	100
10	9.5	95
20	19	95
20	20	100
40	38	95
40	39	98
Urine		
10	10	100
10	10	100
20	20	100
20	20	100
40	39	98
40	39	98

[a] Single determinations; recovery is based on taking the standard through the complete procedure.

Analytical variables. Analytical recovery of ethchlorvynol added to serum and urine (Table 1) was essentially 98% throughout the concentration range studied.

The absorbance at 510 nm follows Beer's Law up to ethchlorvynol concentrations of 100 mg/L; samples with greater concentrations must be diluted with water and reassayed.

Of the various drugs subjected to the method (Table 2) none except phenazopyridine (Pyridium) interfered. To differentiate between the pink color from phenazopyridine and ethchlorvynol in urine or gastric contents by this method (7), mix the final solution (step 5 of the *Qualitative Screening Procedure*) with chloroform, depending on the intensity of the solution: the more intense the color, the greater the volume of chloroform. If ethchlorvynol is the drug present, the pink color will go into the chloroform layer; if phenazopyridine is present, the color will remain in the aqueous layer. Other differences are that phenazopyridine colors the urine orange or red and ethchlorvynol often imparts its distinct odor to gastric specimens.

The day-to-day precision (CV) of this method is 6% for a mean concentration of 20 mg/L.

The sensitivity of the method for ethchlorvynol in serum is 1 mg/L.

Table 2. Drugs Not Reacting in This Method for Ethchlorvynol

Drug	Concn tested, mg/L
Acetaminophen (Tylenol)	100
Amitriptyline hydrochloride (Elavil)	100
Amobarbital, sodium	100
Amphetamine, sulfate	100
Bromide, sodium	2500
Butabarbital, sodium	100
Chloral hydrate	200
Chlordiazepoxide (Librium)	100
Chlorpheniramine maleate (Chlortrimeton)	120
Chlorpromazine hydrochloride (Thorazine)	200
Cocaine hydrochloride	20
Codeine sulfate	20
Demerol hydrochloride	100
Diazepam (Valium)	100
Diphenylhydramine hydrochloride (Benadryl)	100
Flurazepam hydrochloride (Dalmane)	100
Glutethimide (Doriden)	100
Hydromorphone hydrochloride (Dilaudid)	20
Imipramine hydrochloride (Tofranil)	100
Meprobamate	200
Methadone hydrochloride	20
Methaqualone (Sopor)	100
Methdilazine hydrochloride	100
Methyprylon (Noludar)	200
Morphine hydrochloride	20
Nalorphine hydrochloride (Nalline)	100
Pentazocine hydrochloride (Talwin)	100
Perphenazine (Trilafon)	100
Phenobarbital, sodium	200
Phenytoin (Dilantin)	100
Procainamide hydrochloride	100
Prochlorperazine edisylate (Compazine)	200
Promazine hydrochloride (Sparine)	100
Promethazine hydrochloride (Phenergan)	100
Propoxyphene hydrochloride (Darvon)	100
Salicylate, sodium	1500
Secobarbital, sodium	100
Strychnine sulfate	100
Sulfanilamide	1000
Thiopropazate hydrochloride	100
Thioridazine hydrochloride (Mellaril)	100
Trifluoperazine dihydrochloride (Stelazine)	200
Trimethobenzamide hydrochloride (Tigan)	250

Note: Evaluator C. H. Q. notes that some urine samples will turn various shades of blue after reaction with the color reagent. This blue color may visually obscure the pink color formed between ethchlorvynol and the color reagent. Scanning these blue solutions spectrophotometrically will show a peak at 510-515 nm if ethchlorvynol is present.

References

1. Algeri EJ, Katsas GG, Luongo MA. Determination of ethchlorvynol in biologic mediums, and report of two fatal cases. *Am J Clin Pathol* **38**, 125-130 (1962).
2. Wallace JE, Wilson WJ, Dahl EV. A rapid and specific method for determining ethchlorvynol. *J Forens Sci* **9**, 342-352 (1964).
3. Robinson DW. Method for determining ethchlorvynol in urine and serum by gas chromatography. *J Pharm Sci* **57**, 185-186 (1968).
4. Weinberg SB, Dal Cortivo LA. Critique forensic pathology check sample no. FP-47. Commission on Continuing Education, Am. Soc. Clin. Pathol., Chicago, IL, 1969.
5. Frings CS, Cohen PS. Colorimetric method for the quantitative determination of ethchlorvynol (Placidyl) in serum and urine. *Am J Clin Pathol* **54**, 833-836 (1970).
6. Frings CS, Cohen PS. Ethchlorvynol ("Placidyl"): Determination in serum and urine. *Stand Methods Clin Chem* **7**, 209-213 (1972).
7. Frings CS, Queen CA. Elimination of interference by phenazopyridine hydrochloride ("Pyridium") in determining ethchlorvynol ("Placidyl"). *Clin Chem* **19**, 1087 (1973). Letter.

Ethylene Glycol by Gas-Liquid Chromatography

Submitters: William H. Porter and Linda D. Dorie, *Department of Pathology, University of Kentucky Medical Center, Lexington, KY 40536*

Evaluators: C. Andrew Robinson, Jr., and Catherine H. Ketchum, *Department of Pathology, Division of Clinical Pathology, The University of Alabama in Birmingham, Birmingham, AL 35294*

E. Howard Taylor, *Department of Pathology, University of Arkansas for Medical Sciences, Little Rock, AR 72205*

Introduction

Ethylene glycol intoxication is a major clinical emergency that requires prompt identification of the toxic agent so that appropriate therapeutic measures can be instituted (1,2). The toxicity of ethylene glycol is associated with its metabolism by liver alcohol dehydrogenase (EC 1.1.1.1) to several products, including glycolic and oxalic acids; metabolic acidosis ensues, along with damage to renal and cerebral organs (1,2). An effective therapy is to administer ethanol to competitively inhibit the alcohol dehydrogenase-mediated metabolism of ethylene glycol. Hemodialysis and forced diuresis may also be combined with ethanol infusion (3,4).

Because of the short half-life (3 h) of ethylene glycol and because of its highly lethal potential, the toxicology laboratory must provide rapid and reliable determinations of this analyte to assist not only the diagnosis, but also the monitoring of the course of therapy.

Principle

Ethylene glycol reacts with phenylboronic acid to form a cyclic phenylboronate ester (Figure 1), which is quantified by gas-liquid chromatography (5). The internal standard, 1,3-propanediol, forms a six-membered cyclic phenylboronate ester with phenylboronic acid.

Materials and Methods

Reagents

1. *Ethylene glycol stock standard, 2.00 g/L:* Dilute 100 mg of ethylene glycol (99+%; Aldrich Chemical Co., Inc., Milwaukee WI 53233) to volume in a 50-mL volumetric flask, using an aqueous solution of 70 g of bovine serum albumin (BSA, Cohn Fraction V; Sigma Chemical Co., St. Louis, MO 63178) per liter. Aliquots are stable for at least four months if stored frozen. Prepare additional standards of 1.00 and 0.50 g/L, as needed, by appropriate dilution of the stock standard with the BSA solution.
2. *Internal standard:* 1,3-Propanediol (Eastman Organic Chemicals, Rochester, NY 14650), 750 mg/L in acetonitrile. Stable for at least two months when stored refrigerated.
3. *Phenylboronic acid reagent:* Dissolve 5.00 g (41 mmol) of phenylboronic acid per liter of 2,2-dimethoxypropane (both from Aldrich Chemical Co.), which also contains 20 mL of glacial acetic acid per liter. Prepare fresh reagent each day of analysis.

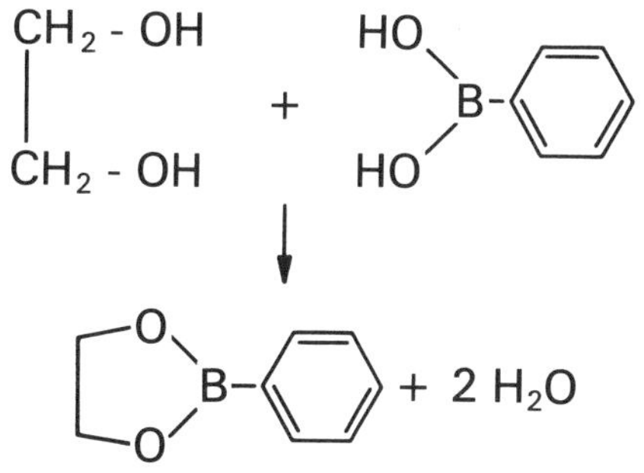

Fig. 1. Reaction of ethylene glycol with phenylboronic acid to form the cyclic phenylboronate ester

Apparatus

1. *Gas chromatograph:* We used a gas chromatograph equipped with a flame ionization detector and an 185 cm × 2 mm (i.d.) silanized glass column packed with 3% OV-1 on 80/100 mesh Supelcoport (Supelco, Bellefonte, PA 16823). The operating temperatures are: column 115 °C, injector 250 °C, detector 300 °C. Gas-flow rates are adjusted to: nitrogen (carrier gas), 30 mL/min; hydrogen, 30 mL/min; air, 240 mL/min.
2. *Recorder:* 10 mV full-scale; chart speed = 0.5 cm/min.

Procedure

1. To 12-mL conical centrifuge tubes add 100 μL of each standard and patient's sample.
2. Add 200 μL of internal standard; vortex-mix.
3. Centrifuge for 5 min in a table-top centrifuge to remove precipitated protein.
4. Transfer 100 μL of the supernate into a 13 × 100 mm Teflon-lined screw-capped test tube, add 100 μL of phenylboronic acid, and vortex-mix.
5. Inject 0.5 to 1.0 μL of the reaction mixture into the gas chromatograph.

Calculations

Measure the ratio of the peak height for ethylene glycol relative to that for the internal standard. Plot the peak height ratio vs the concentration of the standards and determine the concentration of ethylene glycol in the patient's specimen from the standard curve. Alternatively, calculate the concentration of the unknown by linear regression analysis with a hand-held calculator.

Results and Discussion

Analytical Considerations

The chromatographic response for ethylene glycol phenylboronate and the phenylboronate derivative of 1,2-propanediol and 1,3-propanediol is illustrated in Figure 2. The phenylboronate derivatives form rapidly and demonstrate good chromatographic characteristics.

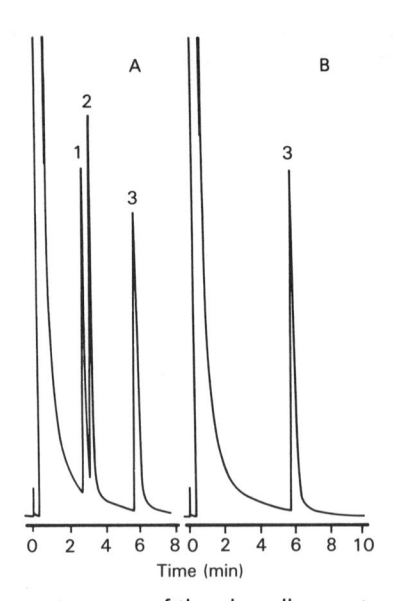

Fig. 2. Chromatograms of the phenylboronates of ethylene glycol (1), 1,2-propanediol (2), and 1,3-propanediol (3)

A, Standard in BSA; B, serum specimen containing no ethylene glycol. The concentration of ethylene glycol in the BSA standard is 1.02 g/L, propylene glycol 1.10 g/L. The concentration of internal standard (3) is 0.75 g/L

The recovery of ethylene glycol from serum samples is approximately 85% of that recovered from aqueous standards. Therefore, the standards must be prepared in an albumin solution to compensate for the amount of ethylene glycol apparently bound to protein. When the assay was standardized in this manner, the analytical recovery of ethylene glycol from pooled serum averaged 97% (range 95-101%) over the concentration range of 0.25 to 5.00 g/L (Table 1). This recovery is not improved by increasing the albumin concentration to 80 g/L and is decreased only slightly (mean 96%) when the albumin concentration is decreased to 50 g/L.

Table 1. Analytical Recovery Studies

	Ethylene glycol, g/L	Mean recovery (and range), %
Evaluators		
C.A.R. and C.H.K.	0.10, 0.50	103.5 (98-109)
E.H.T.	0.50, 2.0	99.3 (96.9-101.6)
Submitters	0.25 - 5.0	97.0 (95-101)

The method demonstrates good precision: within-day CVs are generally <5% over the concentration range of 0.10 to 2.00 g/L (Table 2). The range over which assay response varies linearly with concentration extends to at least 5.00 g/L. If a patient's specimen needs to be diluted, dilute with bovine serum albumin (70 g/L). The lower limit of detection is 10 mg/L.

Using 2,2-dimethoxypropane as the solvent for phenylboronic acid reduces the total water content of the sample injected onto the chromatographic column.

Table 2. Precision Studies

	Ethylene glycol, mg/L			
	Mean	SD	CV, %	n
Within-day precision				
Evaluators				
C.A.R. and C.H.K.	133	15.9	11.9	20
	485	14.5	3.0	20
E.H.T.	512	9.0	1.8	4
	1909	69.0	3.6	4
Submitters	91	4.4	4.8	10
	1014	26.4	2.2	10
Between-day precision				
Evaluators				
C.A.R. and C.H.K.	102	24.0	23.5	30
E.H.T.	508	29.0	5.7	12[a]
	1938	93.0	4.8	12[a]
Submitters	102	6.5	6.3	20
	1010	47.5	4.7	20

[a] Combined within-day and between-day precision (four replicates per day × three days).

Ordinarily immiscible with water, 2,2-dimethoxypropane in the presence of hydrogen ions undergoes acid-catalyzed solvolysis with an equimolar quantity of water to form methanol and acetone in a molar ratio of 2/1 (6). Generally, the phenylboronic acid provides sufficient hydrogen ions to catalyze this reaction. However, freshly opened bottles of phenylboronic acid may contain a high proportion of phenylboronic acid anhydride and thus be an inadequate source of hydrogen ions. Use of this reagent may result in a heterogeneous mixture when mixed with the acetonitrile-precipitated supernate of the sample and may lead to erratic analytical results. To avoid this problem, we routinely add glacial acetic acid to the phenylboronic acid solution.

Ethylene glycol may accumulate on the column or in the injection port and lead to a small amount of sample carryover—i.e., injecting a blank sample after a sample with a high concentration of ethylene glycol may result in a small ethylene glycol response for the blank. The amount of carryover after a 2.0 g/L standard was always <30 mg/L (mean, 13 mg/L; range 5-25 mg/L). This carryover could be eliminated by increasing the column temperature to 275 °C for 10 min after the standard had been injected.

Note: Evaluator E. H. T. observed <50 mg/L carryover after a 2.0 g/L standard. This carryover could be reduced to <10 mg/L by increasing the column temperature to 250 °C for 4 min between injections.

Note: Excess phenylboronic acid also accumulates on the column and might conceivably affect chromatographic determinations of other drugs to be performed on the same column. This accumulated phenylboronic acid may be removed, if desired, by increasing the column temperature to 300 °C for 15 to 20 min. To test for removal of phenylboronic acid, inject a sample of ethylene glycol in acetonitrile. No peak for ethylene glycol should result if the accumulated phenylboronic acid has been removed. Evaluators C. A. R. and C. H. K. found that a longer period of heating at 300 °C may be required to remove accumulated phenylboronic acid. We stress that accumulation of phenylboronic acid has not as yet been proved to cause problems.

Clinical Uses

The estimated 3-h half-life of ethylene glycol in humans was prolonged to 17 h after oral ethanol administration, with therapeutic ethanol concentrations in blood maintained between 1.30 and 2.00 g/L (3). The short half-life of ethylene glycol should be considered when interpreting values for concentrations of ethylene glycol in serum. These concentrations decline precipitously within 24 h of ingestion (2). Therefore, relatively low serum concentrations may be observed even during instances of serious intoxication if several hours have elapsed between the time of ingestion and the time the specimen is collected. Measurement of ethylene glycol in urine may be helpful in documenting ingestion, because significant quantities of ethylene glycol are eliminated by the kidney, and its concentration in urine generally exceeds that in serum (2,3).

Blood concentrations associated with deaths from ethylene glycol intoxication have ranged from 0.30 to 4.30 g/L (7). On the other hand, two patients with initial serum concentrations of ethylene glycol of 6.50 (3) and 5.60 g/L (4) both survived, as a result of early and aggressive therapy with ethanol infusion and hemodialysis. These cases illustrate the importance of the early recognition of the intoxicating agent involved and further indicate that ethylene glycol itself is relatively nontoxic as compared with its acidic metabolites.

Comparison with Other Techniques

Measurement of ethylene glycol by colorimetric (8) and fluorometric (9) procedures, based on its oxidation to formaldehyde, is considered nonspecific. Problems of nonspecificity are also associated with enzymic methods involving alcohol dehydrogenase (10). Among the gas-chromatographic procedures proposed for determining ethylene glycol in serum or blood, those that involve the direct determination of underivatized ethylene glycol suffer from low sensitivity and problems associated with peak tailing (11,12); others, based on derivatization of ethylene glycol, are either tedious and suffer from poor precision (13) or do not provide for the use of an internal standard and have only moderate limits of detection (14). A "high-performance" liquid-chromatographic method (15), based on formation of the benzoyl ester of ethylene glycol, appears to be more complicated and time consuming than the gas-chromatographic procedure described here, may not be as precise, and has not yet been documented to be free from interference by propylene glycol (1,2-propanediol).

The procedure we have described is rapid and simple to perform, has a wide linear dynamic range, demonstrates good precision, and involves a column in general use in many toxicology laboratories. There is no interference from clinically significant concentrations of acetone, ethanol, methanol, isopropanol, amobarbital, butabarbital, pentobarbital, phenobarbital, secobarbital, chlordiazepoxide, diazepam, glutethimide, meprobamate, methaqualone, methyprylon, or phenytoin. Importantly, propylene glycol (1,2-propanediol) and ethylene glycol are well resolved on the OV-1 column, in contrast to their lack of resolution on an OV-17 column (5). Because propylene glycol (400 mL/L) is used as a vehicle for the intravenous administration of diazepam, phenytoin, and other drugs, procedures for determining ethylene glycol must not be susceptible to interference from propylene glycol (16).

References

1. Winek CL, Shingleton DP, Shanor SP. Ethylene and diethylene glycol toxicity. *Clin Toxicol* **13**, 297-324 (1978).
2. Parry MF, Wallach R. Ethylene glycol poisoning. *Am J Med* **57**, 143-150 (1974).
3. Peterson CD, Collins AJ, Himes JM, et al. Ethylene glycol poisoning: Pharmacokinetics during therapy with ethanol and hemodialysis. *N Engl J Med* **304**, 21-23 (1981).
4. Stokes JB, Aueron F. Prevention of organ damage in massive ethylene glycol ingestion. *J Am Med Assoc* **243**, 2065-2066 (1980).
5. Porter WH, Auansakul A. Gas-chromatographic determination of ethylene glycol in serum. *Clin Chem* **28**, 75-78 (1982).
6. Critchfield FE, Bishop ET. Water determination by reaction with 2,2-dimethoxypropane. *Anal Chem* **33**, 1034-1035 (1961).
7. Baselt RC. *Disposition of Toxic Drugs and Chemicals in Man*, 2nd ed., Biomedical Publications, Davis, CA, 1982, p 318.
8. Rajagopal G, Ramakrishman S. A new method for estimation of ethylene glycol in biological material. *Anal Biochem* **65**, 132-136 (1975).
9. Meola JM, Rosano TG, Swift TA. Fluorometry of ethylene glycol in serum. *Clin Chem* **26**, 1709 (1980).
10. Eckfeldt JH, Light RT. Kinetic ethylene glycol assay with use of yeast alcohol dehydrogenase. *Clin Chem* **26**, 1278-1280 (1980).
11. Jain NC, Forney R Jr. Ethylene glycol. In *Methodology for Analytical Toxicology*, I Sunshine, Ed., CRC Press, Inc., West Palm Beach, FL, 1975, pp 165-166.
12. Bost RO, Sunshine I. Ethylene glycol analysis by gas chromatography. *J Anal Toxicol* **4**, 102-103 (1980).
13. Peterson RL, Rodgerson DO. Gas-chromatographic determination of ethylene glycol in serum. *Clin Chem* **20**, 820-824 (1974).
14. Robinson DW, Reive DS. A gas-chromatographic procedure for quantitation of ethylene glycol in postmortem blood. *J Anal Toxicol* **5**, 69-72 (1981).
15. Gupta RN, Eng F, Gupta ML. Liquid-chromatographic determination of ethylene glycol in plasma. *Clin Chem* **28**, 32-33 (1982).
16. Robinson CA Jr, Scott JW, Ketchum C. Propylene glycol interference with ethylene glycol procedures. *Clin Chem* **29**, 727 (1983). Letter.

Iron in Serum by Colorimetry

Submitter: Charles A. Bradley, *Department of Pathology, Vanderbilt University, Nashville, TN*

Evaluator: Kenneth E. Blick, *University of Oklahoma College of Medicine, Oklahoma City, OK 73190*

Introduction

Iron, the most abundant of the trace elements in the human body, is believed to be essential for all living cells. It participates in a variety of vital processes, from cellular oxidative mechanisms to the transport of oxygen to the tissues (*1*). Of the total amount of iron in an adult (4 to 5 g), about 70 to 75% is actively in use in vital physiological roles, the remaining 25 to 30% being present in various storage forms that can be readily mobilized if necessary (*2*). The physiologically active iron is present mainly in oxygen-carrying chromoproteins such as hemoglobin (65%) and myoglobin (3 to 5%), and in various enzymes such as the cytochromes, cytochrome oxidase, peroxidase, and catalase.

In food such as liver and meat, iron is present in the trivalent (ferric) form conjugated to protein. To be absorbed by humans, it must be separated from the protein and reduced to the ferrous (bivalent) form. Both of these processes take place in the stomach and the small intestine, being promoted by ascorbic acid in foods and by gastric acids and being delayed in the presence of pancreatic juice, phosphates, and phytates (*3*). Physiologically, iron absorption depends on the volume of stored iron and on the erythropoietic activity of the bone marrow. The absorbed iron is carried across the mucosal cell membranes by the protein apoferritin (relative molecular mass 460 000), which, when combined with iron, is called ferritin (*4*). From the mucosal cells, iron is delivered to the plasma, where, in the trivalent form, it is covalently bound with a specific iron-transport protein, transferrin (*5*) (Figure 1). This protein, which by electrophoresis is shown to be a β_1-globulin, is ordinarily 20 to 50% saturated with iron, the saturation being greatest in the morning and least in the evening. Most of the iron in plasma is transported to the bone marrow for synthesis of hemoglobin. Smaller quantities of iron are deposited in storage organs such as the liver, spleen, and bone marrow. Very small amounts are excreted in the urine and feces. If the concentrations of iron in serum decrease, almost all iron is directed toward erythropoiesis; when the concentrations increase, more iron is diverted to the storage organs.

Unlike other trace elements, iron hemostasis is regulated primarily by absorption and not by excretion. Because only small amounts of iron are excreted from the body, the absorption of iron from the intestine must be controlled so that it does not accumulate in tissue to toxic concentrations. An abundance of iron in the tissues—which indicates that the intake of iron exceeds the capacity of the body to excrete it—can result from either of two situations (*6*): an abnormality of the control mechanism for the intestinal absorption of iron, so that more iron is absorbed than the body requires; or an iron intake so great that it overwhelms the regulatory system of absorption in an otherwise normal individual.

Because iron absorption is generally well regulated, toxicity is not a common problem. However, the accidental ingestion of excess iron is an important cause of death in children, ranking second only to salicylates as a cause of death from drug overdose in childhood (*7*). Indeed, before the use of the chelating agent deferoxamine, the death rate in children from iron intoxication exceeded that from acetylsalicylic acid (*8*). The widespread use of ferrous sulfate for treating iron-deficiency anemia has increased the opportunity for accidental iron poisoning, and the coloring and candy-coating of ferrous sulfate tablets make them appealing to small children. Besides treatment with deferoxamine, early identification of iron as the poisoning agent has helped improve the chances for recovery of patients suffering from iron intoxication. The development of rapid, accurate methods for measuring the concentration of iron in serum has aided the timely diagnosis and treatment of iron toxicity.

Principle

Iron in serum is usually measured colorimetrically. First the iron is separated from transferrin by strong acid. Next the reduced iron reacts with a chromogen to produce an iron-chromogen complex. Various chromogenic compounds have been evaluated for this use (*9*). Ferrozine [3-(2-pyridyl)-5,6-bis(4-phenylsulfonic acid)-1,2,4-triazine] forms a water-soluble magenta complex with iron (*10*) and has been used in iron determinations (*9,11*). The Ferrozine method originally described by Persijn et al. (*11*) requires only 0.5 mL of serum and avoids the need for protein precipitation; it forms the basis for the procedure presented here.

At an acid pH and in the presence of a reducing agent, transferrin-bound iron in serum dissociates to form ferrous ions. The ferrous ions react with Ferrozine to form a magenta complex with an absorption maximum near 560 nm. The difference in color intensity at 560 nm, before and after adding Ferrozine, is proportional to the concentration of iron.

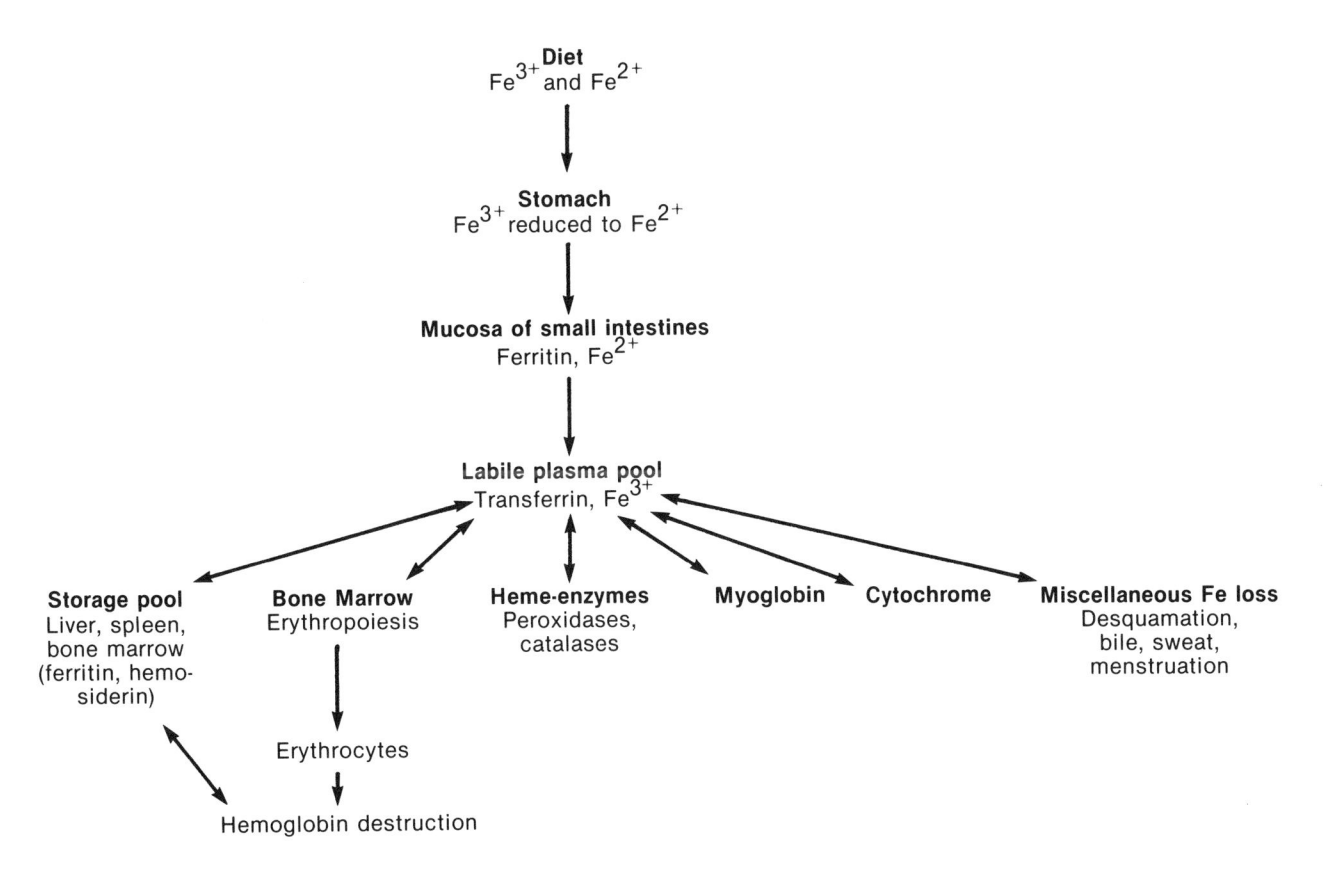

Fig. 1. Schematic diagram of iron metabolism

Materials and Methods

Collection and Handling of Specimens

All materials used in the collection and storage of blood should be iron-free. Serum should be separated from the erythrocytes as soon as the blood clots, to avoid hemolysis. Hemolyzed samples cannot be used because each milligram of hemoglobin contains 3.4 µg of iron. At least 0.5 mL of serum is required for each determination. Samples should be analyzed within four days when stored at room temperature (25 °C), or within one week when stored refrigerated (4 °C).

Materials

The reagents used in this procedure were purchased from the Sigma Chemical Co., St. Louis, MO. However, these reagents are not unique and may be obtained from other manufacturers.

1. *Iron buffer reagent* (cat. no. 565-1): hydroxylamine hydrochloride, 15 g/L in acetate buffer (0.7 mol/L, pH 4.5). This reagent also contains a surfactant and should be stored at 4 °C.
2. *Iron color reagent* (cat. no. 565-3): Ferrozine, 8.5 g/L in hydroxylamine hydrochloride solution (reagent 1). A stabilizer is also included; this reagent is stored at 4 °C when not in use.
3. *Iron standard* (cat. no. 565-5): iron, 5.0 mg/L (89 µmol/L), in hydroxylamine hydrochloride. The standard is stored at room temperature.
4. Disposable polyethylene cuvettes (Evergreen Scientific, Los Angeles, CA; cat. no. 3125B) were used as the reaction vessels for the iron assay.

Procedure

1. Label four or more of the disposable polyethylene cuvettes as follows: blank, standard, control, and test$_1$ ... test$_N$.
2. Add 2.5 mL of iron buffer reagent to all cuvettes.
3. Pipet 0.5 mL of iron-free water into the cuvette labeled "blank," 0.5 mL of iron standard into the cuvette labeled "standard," and 0.5 mL of control or serum into the respective "control" or "test" cuvettes. Cap all cuvettes and mix by inversion.
4. Read the absorbance (initial A) of the standard, control(s), and test(s) against the blank in a spectrophotometer at 560 nm.
5. Add 50 µL of iron color reagent to all cuvettes, cap, and mix by inversion.
6. Incubate all samples at 37 °C for 10 min.
7. Read the absorbance (final A) of the standard, control(s), and test(s) against the blank in a spectrophotometer at 560 nm.
8. Calculate results as follows:

$$\text{Total iron concn (mg/L)} = 5 \times \frac{\text{Final } A_{test} - \text{initial } A_{test}}{\text{Final } A_{std} - \text{initial } A_{std}}$$

Quality Control

Frozen aliquots of serum pools or commercially available control material are suitable controls for this procedure.

Note: Contamination is a major problem with any trace-element analysis. Therefore, plastic disposable pipettes and pipette tips should be used in the procedure and discarded after use. Glass pipettes may be used, but they will require acid washing and rinsing with iron-free water before use in the iron assay.

Results and Discussion

At birth, the average concentration of iron in serum approaches 2.00 mg/L, but decreases rapidly within hours to less than 0.50 mg/L; concentrations then increase to normal adult values after the first three weeks of life. In adults, iron in serum is normally 0.60 to 1.50 mg/L for men and 0.50 to 1.30 mg/L for women. Serum concentrations of iron in the elderly decrease to 0.40 to 0.80 mg/L (2).

Although iron is an essential trace element necessary for all living cells within the human body, excess iron may be toxic and, in sufficient quantities, fatal. Large doses of iron are usually well tolerated by adults; however, a relatively few iron tablets may cause death in children. Signs and symptoms of toxicity, which may occur as early as 30 min after ingestion or may be delayed several hours, include gastrointestinal irritation and abdominal pain, often accompanied by vomiting and bloody diarrhea. After 16 to 24 h the patient may develop severe metabolic acidosis, cyanosis, drowsiness, lethargy, convulsions, circulatory collapse, coma, and death. If the patient survives the first few hours, a transient, nearly asymptomatic period may precede death. Patients who recover may still have severe scarring from corrosive injury to the gastrointestinal tract.

Although the mechanisms leading to the clinical signs and symptoms of iron intoxication are not clearly understood, they are related to the presence in the circulatory systems of excess unbound iron, and do not occur unless the concentration of iron exceeds the serum iron-binding capacity. In normal, healthy individuals the serum iron-binding capacity is 2.50-4.00 mg/L (44.8-71.6 μmol/L). Shock and coma may occur in up to 50% of patients whose serum concentrations of iron exceed 7.00 mg/L (125 μmol/L) (12). Concentrations greater than 5.00 mg/L (89.5 μmol/L) indicate serious poisoning (13).

Treatment of iron toxicity has been primarily with the chelating agent deferoxamine, a sideramine derived from *Actinomycetacea*. Deferoxamine has been useful in treating acute iron poisoning in children, 100 mg of deferoxamine combining with 9.3 mg of trivalent iron to remove it from transferrin, hemosiderin, and ferritin via excretion in urine (14). Deferoxamine forms a nontoxic, unabsorbable complex with iron in the intestinal tract and competes for the iron of ferritin and hemosiderin in the tissues; it partly removes the iron from transferrin, but the iron in cytochromes and hemoglobin is unaffected. Because deferoxamine itself is potentially toxic, it should be administered only after acute iron intoxication has been clearly documented. Use of a rapid, reliable method for measuring iron concentrations in patients with acute iron poisoning is of obvious value in establishing the management regimen for these individuals.

References

1. Woo J, Trevting JJ, Cannon DC. In *Clinical Diagnosis and Management by Laboratory Methods*. 16th ed., JB Henry, Ed., WB Saunders Co., Philadelphia, PA, 1979, pp 294-298.
2. Tietz NW. Blood gases and electrolytes. In *Fundamentals of Clinical Chemistry*, 2nd ed., WB Saunders Co., Philadelphia, PA, 1976, pp 922-929.
3. Jacobs A, Rhodes J, Peters DK, et al. Gastric acidity and iron absorption. *Br J Haematol* **12**, 728-735 (1966).
4. Wheby MS, Crosby WH. The gastrointestinal tract and iron absorption. *Blood* **22**, 416-428, (1963).
5. Bauer JD, Ackermann PG, Toro G. *Clinical Laboratory Methods*, 8th ed., CV Mosby Co., St. Louis, MO, 1974, pp 119-127.
6. Sims FH. Pathologic processes. In *Applied Biochemistry of Clinical Disorders*, AG Gornall, Ed., Harper and Row, Hagerstown, MD, 1980, pp 24-25.
7. Hill JD. Pediatric clinical biochemistry. *Ibid.*, pp 363-367.
8. Sisson TRC. Acute iron poisoning in children. *Q Rev Pediatr* **15**, 47-49 (1960).
9. Carter P. Spectrophotometric determination of serum iron at the submicrogram level with a new reagent (Ferrozine). *Anal Biochem* **40**, 450-458, 1971.
10. Stookey LL. A new spectrophotometric reagent for iron. *Anal Chem* **42**, 779-781 (1970).
11. Persijn JP, van der Slik W, Riethorst A. Determination of serum iron and latent iron-binding capacity (LIBC). *Clin Chim Acta* **35**, 91-98 (1971).
12. Dreisback RH. *Handbook of Poisoning. Prevention, Diagnosis, and Treatment*, 10th ed., Lange Medical Publications, Los Altos, CA, 1980.
13. Callender ST. Treatment of iron deficiency. In *Iron in Biochemistry and Medicine*, A Jacobs, M Worwood, Eds., Academic Press, London, 1974, pp 540-541.
14. Vaughan VC, McKay JR, Nelson WE. (Eds.) *Textbook of Pediatrics*, 10th ed., WB Saunders Co., Philadelphia, PA, 1974, p 1673.

Lead in Whole Blood by Flameless Atomic Absorption Spectrophotometry

Submitter: Roger L. Boeckx, *Department of Laboratory Medicine, Children's Hospital National Medical Center, and Department of Child Health and Development, George Washington University School of Medicine and Health Sciences, Washington, DC 20010*

Evaluator: John T. McCall, *Mayo Clinic, Rochester, MN 55905*

Introduction

Lead poisoning continues to be a significant public health problem. Despite more aggressive safety measures, industrial exposure is still a frequent cause of work-related illness, and lead poisoning in children, although somewhat improved in recent years, continues as a cause of childhood morbidity.

The effect of urban exposure to lead is indicated in recent studies that show that the concentration of lead in the blood of typical urban residents is perhaps 100-fold the typical concentration in prehistoric times (1). Contemporary studies also show that the mean concentration of lead in blood from an isolated Himalayan population was only 34 µg/L (2), in contrast to the average blood lead concentration in urban children from the Washington, DC, area: 139 (SD 97) µg/L (Boeckx, unpublished data).

The most common sources of exposure include toxic amounts of lead from the paint and plumbing in old houses, dust contaminated by exhaust fumes from automobiles burning leaded gasoline, industrial emissions, and on-the-job exposure in metal-smelting and battery-reclamation industries.

The symptoms of chronic lead poisoning include gastrointestinal disturbance, anemia, insomnia, weight loss, motor weakness, muscle paralysis, and nephropathy.

Some studies (3,4) have indicated that lead may adversely affect the brain at concentrations in blood that are significantly lower than those associated with overt symptoms of lead poisoning. The accurate measurement of lead in blood, even at low concentrations, is essential in evaluating and treating children and adults who have been exposed to excessive amounts of lead.

In the body, lead is distributed in two major pools: a soft-tissue pool, and a skeletal bone pool. While the residence time in the soft-tissue pool is short, approximately 30 days, the residence time in bone can be as long as 30 years. The lead stored in bone is physiologically inert, but tends to reflect the total body burden of lead. Conversely, lead in the soft-tissue pool is responsible for significant toxicity, and reflects recent or current exposure. The concentration of lead in blood represents the concentration of lead in the soft-tissue pool, and as such can be used only to evaluate recent exposure; it is not a reliable measure of the total body burden of lead (1).

Most of the spectrophotometric methods for measuring lead are too tedious, imprecise, and subject to contamination to be useful. Early atomic absorption methods involved direct aspiration techniques that required as much as 10 mL of whole blood, making them unsuitable for use with children. With flameless atomic absorption methods, lead can be measured in 50-µL blood samples, a distinct advantage for measurements in the pediatric population.

Principle

The method described is a modification of the method of Fernandez (5,6). Samples of whole blood are diluted in a detergent solution and transferred into a precisely positioned graphite tube in a graphite furnace. The graphite tube is heated to dry, char, and finally atomize the sample. During the atomizing step, the atomic absorption spectrophotometer records the peak absorbance, which is compared with values on a standard curve prepared by the method of standard additions.

Materials and Methods

Reagents

1. *De-ionized water*: The de-ionized water should be of the highest purity possible, and should have a specific resistance of at least 18 MΩ-cm.

2. *Stock lead standard, 1000 mg/L*: An adequate certified stock standard solution (1000 mg/L) can be purchased from Fisher Scientific Co., Pittsburgh, PA.

3. *Diluted stock standard, 10 mg/L*: Dilute 10 mL of stock lead standard to 1000 mL with de-ionized water.

4. *Whole blood*: Fresh whole blood collected in evacuated specimen tubes containing disodium EDTA is required. The final disodium EDTA concentration should be the same as that in the specimens collected for analysis, i.e., approximately 1.5 mg/mL of whole blood. A total of 50 mL of pooled blood is required to prepare a standard curve. The blood should be well-mixed before use.

5. *Working standards*: Using the utmost precision,

prepare a series of working standards according to the following table:

Concn of standard, µg/L	Volume, mL		
	Diluted stock standard	De-ionized water	Whole blood
x	0	1.0	9.0
x + 200	0.2	0.8	9.0
x + 400	0.4	0.6	9.0
x + 600	0.6	0.4	9.0
x + 800	0.8	0.2	9.0

Add the diluted stock standard and de-ionized water to 10-mL volumetric flasks. Then add blood to the 10-mL mark and mix gently but thoroughly. These working whole-blood standards can be aliquoted and frozen. At −70 °C, they are stable for several months.

6. *Triton X-100 detergent*: Dilute 1 mL of Triton X-100 to 1000 mL with de-ionized water.

Apparatus

All glassware used in this procedure should be washed, soaked overnight in 4 mol/L nitric acid, and rinsed thoroughly with de-ionized water.

For the procedure described here, the Submitter used a Model 603 atomic absorption spectrophotometer fitted with a Model HGA 2100 graphite furnace, a ramp accessory, and a Model AS-1 automatic sampling system (all from Perkin-Elmer Corp., Norwalk, CT). A lead hollow cathode lamp was operated at 10 mA and the absorbance of lead at 283.3 nm was measured. Instrument conditions were as follows:

Slit width	1.0 mm
Purge gas	nitrogen
Gas flow	50 mL/min, interrupted mode
Drying step	110 °C, 40 s; ramp 30 s
Charring step	550 °C, 40 s; ramp 10 s
Atomizing step	2000 °C, 10 s; ramp off
Automatic high temp.	on

Set the autosampler to inject 20-µL samples in triplicate and use the spectrophotometer to record the maximum absorbance reached during the 10-s atomizing period. Deuterium arc background correction is required to eliminate interference. The pyrolytically coated graphite tubes can be used for about 100 firings each. Some lead is lost if charring temperatures exceed 600 °C, and atomizing temperatures above 2000 °C reduce sensitivity.

Collection and Handling of Specimens

Capillary (finger-stick) or venous whole blood can be used. Samples should be collected in trace-metal-free containers with EDTA. For capillary samples, the EDTA-treated collection tubes available from Becton Dickinson, Paramus, NJ 07652, or Sarstedt, Princeton, NJ 08540, are acceptable. A standard plastic syringe and an EDTA-treated evacuated blood-collection tube are acceptable for venipuncture collection. Whole blood collected in heparinized containers cannot be used because heparin interferes with this procedure (7). Samples should be analyzed as soon as possible, but if necessary, they can be stored for as long as one week at 4 °C. Samples should be gently but thoroughly mixed before an aliquot is removed for analysis.

Procedure

Preparation of the standard curve. Because graphite furnace procedures are matrix sensitive, use the method of standard additions to prepare a standard curve, preparing the working standards as described in the *Reagents* section. Use the procedure outlined below to prepare the standard curve.

1. Mix the working standards well, and dilute 50 µL of each of the five working standards (in duplicate) with 200 µL of Triton X-100 solution (1 mL/L). An easily reproducible procedure is to use a precise dispensing device to dispense 200-µL aliquots of the Triton X-100 into plastic cups and then, with a 50-µL pipettor with a plastic tip, transfer 50 µL of well-mixed whole-blood standard into the cup. Rinse the pipette tip five times with the diluent/blood mixture in the cup. Unfortunately, because of the high viscosity of whole blood, automated dilutor-dispensers are not useful.

2. Place Triton X-100 in a plastic cup in the first position of the autosampler tray and use this to adjust the instrument to zero. In the next sample cups, place the five diluted standards in duplicate. Begin the analysis, using the instrument settings described in *Apparatus*.

3. Plot the mean of six absorbance readings for each standard against the amount of added lead in each standard. Figure 1 shows a typical standard curve. Draw the best-fitting straight line through the five points (the *dashed* line in Figure 1). This line will intersect the y-axis at a point above the origin. Draw parallel to the first line a line passing through the origin. This last line (the *solid* line in Figure 1) is the standard curve to use in the assay.

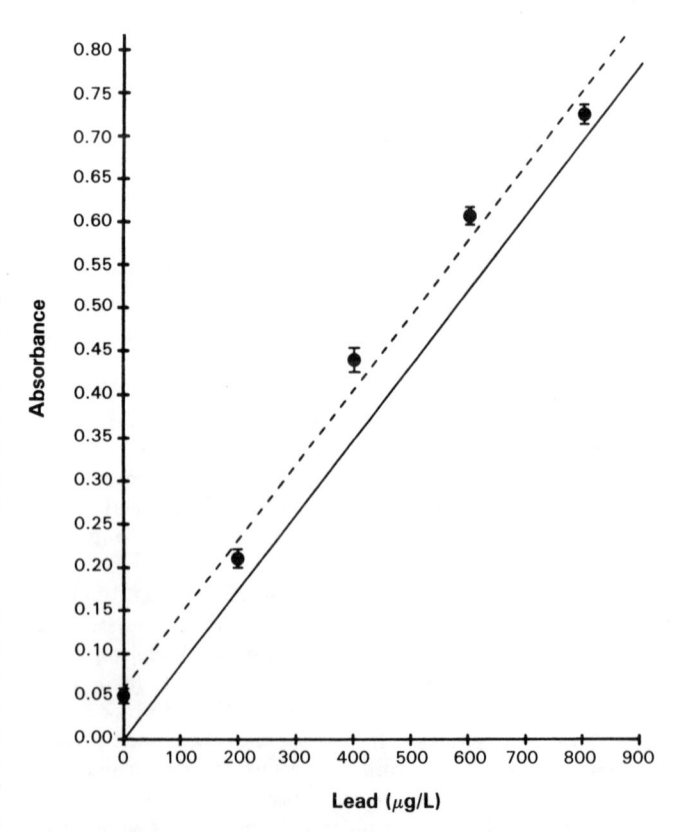

Fig. 1. Sample standard curve using the method of standard additions

Each point is the mean of six absorbance readings. The *bar* around each point defines the mean ± 1 SD range at each concentration. The *dashed line* is the best-fitting straight line through the points. The *solid line*, the actual standard curve used in the assay, is parallel to the dashed line but passes through the origin

This procedure compensates for the lead content of the blood used to prepare the standard solutions. The actual concentration of lead in this blood is the absolute value of the x-intercept of the dashed line—66 µg/L in Figure 1.

Analysis of samples. Dilute and analyze in triplicate well-mixed samples of whole blood as described for the standards above (step 1 above). Compare the mean absorbance with the standard curve to determine the concentration of lead in the blood.

Reference Ranges

Concentrations of lead in blood are usually interpreted in conjunction with the concentration of erythrocyte protoporphyrin (EP) in blood. Because lead inhibits ferrochelatase (EC 4.99.1.1), protoporphyrin IX accumulates in erythrocytes. In lead poisoning, this porphyrin is present in erythrocytes as a zinc chelate—zinc protoporphyrin—and is usually measured by extraction from whole blood with an acidified organic solvent, followed by fluorometry (8,9).

As defined by the Centers for Disease Control (CDC), lead poisoning has occurred when any of the following is true (10):

1. Lead concentrations in two successive blood samples equal or exceed 700 µg/L, with or without symptoms.
2. The concentration of EP equals or exceeds 2500 µg/L and a confirmed concentration of lead in blood equals or exceeds 500 µg/L.
3. A concentration of EP greater than 1099 µg/L is associated with a blood lead concentration of 300 µg/L or more and compatible symptoms.
4. A confirmed concentration of lead in blood greater than 499 µg/L is associated with compatible symptoms and evidence of toxicity—e.g., an abnormal concentration of EP, a positive result for the calcium disodium EDTA mobilization test, or increased urinary excretion of delta-aminolevulinic acid or coproporphyrin.

In addition, the CDC has established the following system of risk classification (10) for assessing the relative risk of lead poisoning in asymptomatic children.

Lead in blood, µg/L	Erythrocyte protoporphyrin, µg/L of whole blood			
	<499	500-1099	1100-2499	>2500
Not measured	I	*	*	*
<299	I	Ia	Ia	EPP[a]
300-499	Ib	II	III	III
500-699	**	III	III	IV
>700	**	**	IV	IV

*Knowledge of blood lead concentration is necessary to estimate risk.
**This combination of results is not usually observed in practice; if they are, the patient should be retested with venous blood as soon as possible.
[a]Erythropoietic protoporphyria.

These various risk classifications can be interpreted as follows:

Class I: The accepted reference range for blood lead in children is less than 300 µg/L. The concentration of EP in healthy children is usually less than 500 µg/L. Therefore, Class I children represent the "normal" child who is at low risk.

Class Ia: The most common cause of increased EP other than lead poisoning is iron-deficiency anemia. Therefore, Class Ia children will usually be found to be iron deficient and are at low risk for lead poisoning.

Class Ib: A slightly increased concentration of lead in blood in the presence of a normal value for EP usually suggests that the blood sample used for the lead determination was contaminated. A fresh sample should be collected and the tests repeated.

Classes II and III: Children in these classes are at risk and should be evaluated for lead poisoning.

Class IV: These children have frank lead poisoning, and should receive immediate treatment and extensive follow-up.

Discussion

To evaluate the accuracy of this method for measuring lead, the Submitter determined the lead content of 15 proficiency specimens prepared by the CDC as part of their blood-lead proficiency testing program. These specimens, samples of bovine blood from animals that had ingested various amounts of lead in their drinking water, have expected values assigned by the CDC based upon analyses by several reference laboratories. The correlation between the expected lead concentration (x) and the result by this procedure (y) is illustrated in Figure 2. The equation of the best-fitting straight line through these 15 points is $y = 1.02x - 20.46$; the correlation coefficient (r) was 0.982, and the standard error of the estimate (S_{yx}) was 33.29.

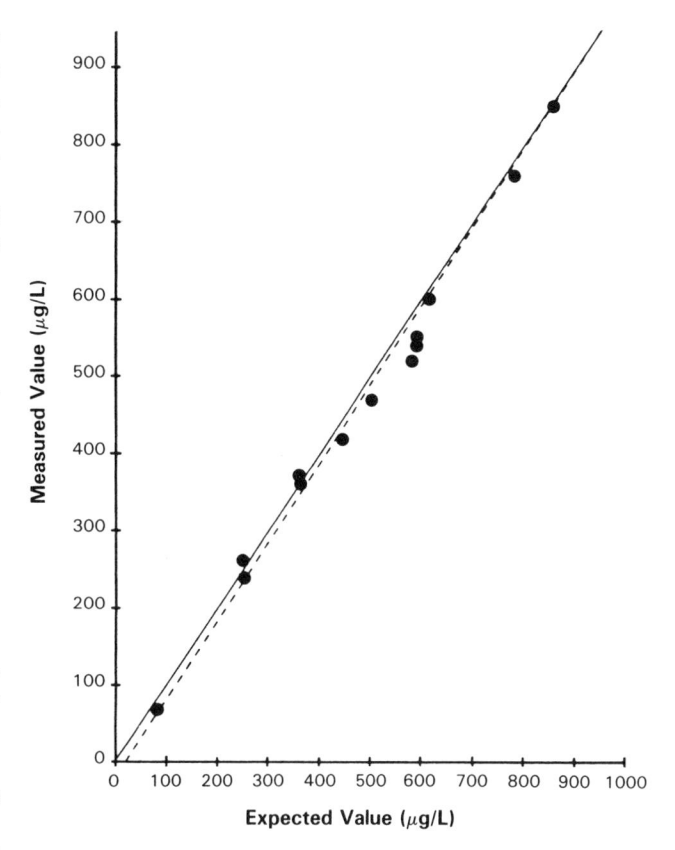

Fig. 2. Comparison of blood results obtained with the flameless atomic absorption method (measured values) and consensus values as reported by the CDC (expected values)
The *dashed line* is the best-fitting straight line through the points. The *solid line* is the line of identity

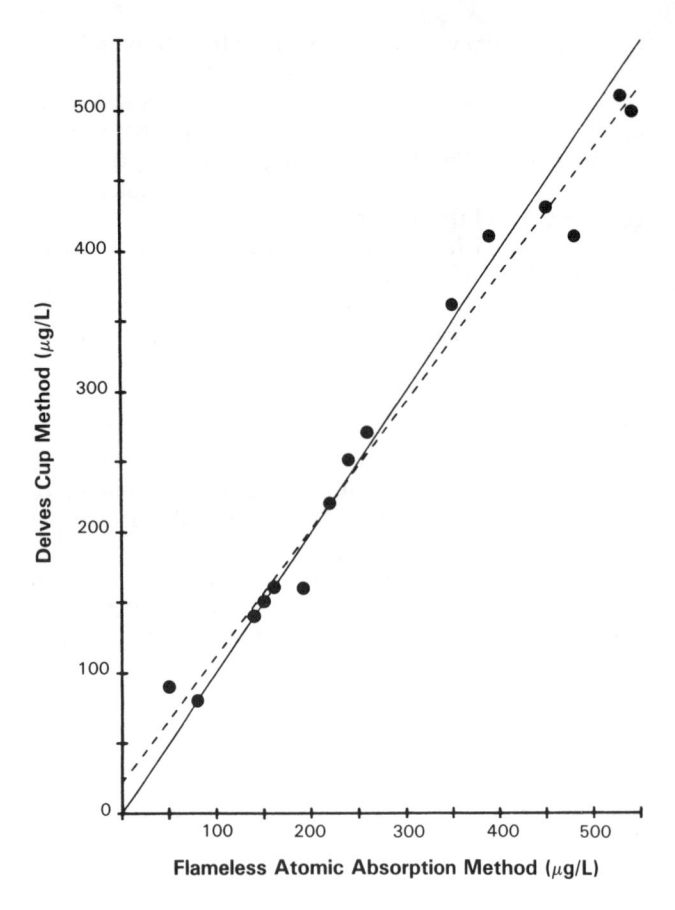

Fig. 3. Comparison of results by the flameless atomic absorption method with those by the Delves cup method

The *dashed line* is the best-fitting straight line through the points. The *solid line* is the line of identity

Table 1. Precision of Lead Determination in Whole Blood

	Within-run (n = 15)		Run-to-run (n = 15)	
Mean, µg/L	190	676	101	550
SD, µg/L	22	41	13	11
CV, %	11.6	6.11	12.9	2.0

Proper alignment of the graphite furnace in the light-beam path of the spectrophotometer is essential for accurate results. Also, correct positioning of the sample probe at insertion is critical: the sample must be placed precisely on the bottom of the graphite tube. Although the analyses can be performed without the use of an autosampler, precision is much better when automatic sample placement is used.

The flameless atomic absorption method for measuring blood lead concentration is a convenient micro-scale procedure that is particularly useful in screening populations of children for lead exposure. The method is accurate and precise, and correlates well with other procedures in current use.

Note: Evaluator J. T. M. obtained consistently lower absorbances for standards prepared in outdated blood samples than for those in fresh blood.

The Submitter also compared results by this method with a Delves cup procedure (6,11). The correlation between these two methods is shown in Figure 3. The best-fitting straight line through these 15 points (Figure 3) is $y = 0.901\,x + 21.80$ ($r = 0.980$, and $S_{yx} = 22.07$).

From the calibration curve shown in Figure 1, an analytical recovery of 100.3% was calculated.

Precision was evaluated by using lead-supplemented whole-blood control materials prepared as described above for the standards. The results of the precision study are summarized in Table 1.

The results of the assay are linear with lead concentrations to 800 µg/L. Samples with greater lead concentrations should be diluted with an equal volume of the lowest concentration calibration standard and re-analyzed.

As with all analytical procedures for measuring the concentration of a trace metal, take special care to avoid sample contamination. When samples are collected by skin puncture, clean the skin carefully. Do not collect the first drop of blood, and make every attempt to avoid direct contact between the collection device and the skin. Highly pure de-ionized water must be used, and glassware must be scrupulously cleaned. A clean, relatively dust-free environment is helpful in avoiding contamination.

The assistance of Mr. Bart Serrano (Department of Human Services, Government of the District of Columbia) in performing the Delves cup analyses is gratefully acknowledged.

References

1. Committee on Lead in the Human Environment. *Lead in the Human Environment*, National Academy of Sciences, Washington, DC, 1980.
2. Piomelli S, Corash L, Corash MB, et al. Blood lead concentrations in a remote Himalayan population. *Science* **210**, 1135-1137 (1980).
3. Needleman HL, Gunnoe C, Leviton A, et al. Deficits in psychologic and classroom performance of children with elevated dentine lead levels. *N Engl J Med* **300**, 689-695 (1974).
4. Charney E. Sub-encephalopathic lead poisoning: Central nervous system effects in children. In *Lead Absorption in Children*, JJ Chisolm Jr, DM O'Hara, Eds., Urban and Schwarzenberg, Baltimore, MD, 1982, pp 35-42.
5. Fernandez FJ. Micromethod for lead determination in whole blood atomic absorption spectrophotometry with use of the graphite furnace. *Clin Chem* **21**, 558-561 (1975).
6. Boeckx RL. Trace metals. In *Pediatric Clinical Chemistry*, JM Hicks, RL Boeckx, Eds., WB Saunders, Philadelphia, PA, 1984, pp 571-600.
7. Evenson MA, Pendergast DD. Rapid ultramicro determination of lead concentration by atomic absorption spectrophotometry, with use of a graphite-tube furnace. *Clin Chem* **20**, 163-171 (1974).
8. Piomelli S. Free erythrocyte porphyrins in the detection of undue absorption of Pb and of Fe deficiency. *Clin Chem* **23**, 264-269 (1977).
9. Labbé RF. Inherited and induced disorders in porphyrin metabolism. *Op. cit.* (ref. 6), pp 548-570.
10. Centers for Disease Control. *Preventing Lead Poisoning in Young Children*, Atlanta, GA, 1978.
11. Delves HT. A micro-sampling method for the rapid determination of lead in blood by atomic absorption spectrophotometry. *Analyst* **95**, 431-438 (1970).

Mercury in Urine by Atomic Absorption Spectrophotometry, with Use of a Mercury Hydride System

Submitter: Jerry L. McHan, *Pathologists' Service, P.A., Atlanta, GA 30302*

Evaluator: Gary L. Smith, *SmithKline Bio-Science Laboratory, Chicago, IL 60195*

Introduction

Mercury, a highly toxic metal, is widely used in medicine, agriculture, and industry, and thus is particularly hazardous. It occurs as the free metal or as organic or inorganic salts. The free metal, e.g., as found in thermometers or barometers, has the least oral toxicity. Organic salts of mercury (used as antiseptics and fungicides) and inorganic salts (antiseptics and pigments) vary in degrees of toxicity, some compounds in each category being highly toxic if taken orally.

The characteristics of mercury poisoning depend on its chemical form and the degree of exposure to it. Symptoms of acute toxicity, usually predominantly gastrointestinal, begin with thirst, nausea with retching, and pain in the pharynx and abdomen and proceed to vomiting of blood-stained material. Later, toxicity manifests as hemorrhagic gastritis and colitis with uremia and circulatory collapse. Patients surviving one to three days develop stomatitis, gastritis, colitis, and severe degeneration of the renal tubules. Death is usually due to irreversible renal failure. In addition, the corrosive preparations of mercury may cause immediate necrosis of the buccal, pharyngeal, and gastrointestinal mucosa.

Chronic intoxication with inorganic mercury compounds results in loosened teeth, gingivitis, and mouth ulcers. Neurological symptoms include mental fatigue, irritability, apprehension, withdrawal, muscle tremors, and slurred speech. Chronic exposure to organic mercury typically affects the central nervous system, causing lesions of the spinal cord.

Although the diagnosis of mercury poisoning must be based on a history of exposure and physical examination, with only a secondary reliance on the concentration of mercury in body fluids, the ability to measure mercury, particularly in urine, is a valuable tool. Moreover, a rapid yet sensitive and precise method for measuring urinary concentrations of mercury is desirable for mass screening of exposed individuals.

Principle

Inorganic and organic compounds of mercury are reduced to elemental mercury by reaction with sodium borohydride under acidic conditions.

$$Hg^{2+} + 2BH_4^- \longrightarrow Hg\uparrow + H_2\uparrow + B_2H_6\uparrow$$
$$\text{gas} \quad \text{gas} \quad \text{gas}$$

The mercury vapor released in this reaction is carried into an absorption cell of an atomic absorption spectrophotometer by an inert carrier gas (nitrogen or argon).

Materials and Methods

Apparatus

The Submitter uses a Model 603 atomic absorption spectrophotometer (Perkin-Elmer Corp., Norwalk, CT) with a mercury-hydride system attachment (MHS-10). An electrode discharge lamp is used as the light source, with the wavelength set at 254.0 nm, slit width at 0.4 cm. Absorbance is monitored with a 10-mV recorder. A schematic representation of the MHS-10 and the gas flow pattern is shown in Figure 1.

The major component of the MHS-10 is a multipath valve operated manually by a plunger. Inert gas (nitrogen or argon) enters the instrument at a pressure of 250 kPa. A built-in pressure reducer, set at 1.5 kPa by the manufacturer, controls the gas flow. Two flow restrictors, F_1 and F_2, and the multipath valve are connected to the outlet of the pressure reducer.

In the standby condition, inert gas flows continuously through inlet P of the multipath valve to outlet A and thence through flow restrictor F_3, which has a nominal flow rate of 650 mL/min. When the reaction flask containing the sample solution is connected to the apparatus, the inert gas stream flows through hose e to the quartz cell, thus purging the system of air. A continuous stream of inert gas flows through restrictor F_1 (nominal flow rate 25 mL/min) and line b to the immersion tube. The flow of gas from the immersion tube, combined with the conical form of the reaction flask, mixes the solution thoroughly. A third stream of inert gas flows through restrictor F_2 (nominal flow rate 400 mL/min) and line a to the reaction flask. The total nominal flow rate in the standby condition is about 1100 mL/min.

To measure the mercury in a sample, push the plunger of the MHS-10 down and hold it down. This shuts off the gas stream through F_3 and applies pressure from outlet B of the valve to the reductant reservoir via line c. Reductant, forced through hose d into the immersion tube, is then transported into the sample solution and mixed thoroughly by the violent reaction and the formation of hydrogen gas after the reaction. The metallic mercury vapor is transported to the quartz cell, where the intensity of its absorption is measured.

When the tracing on the chart recorder indicates that the absorbance has peaked and is beginning to decrease, release the plunger. This stops the flow of reductant

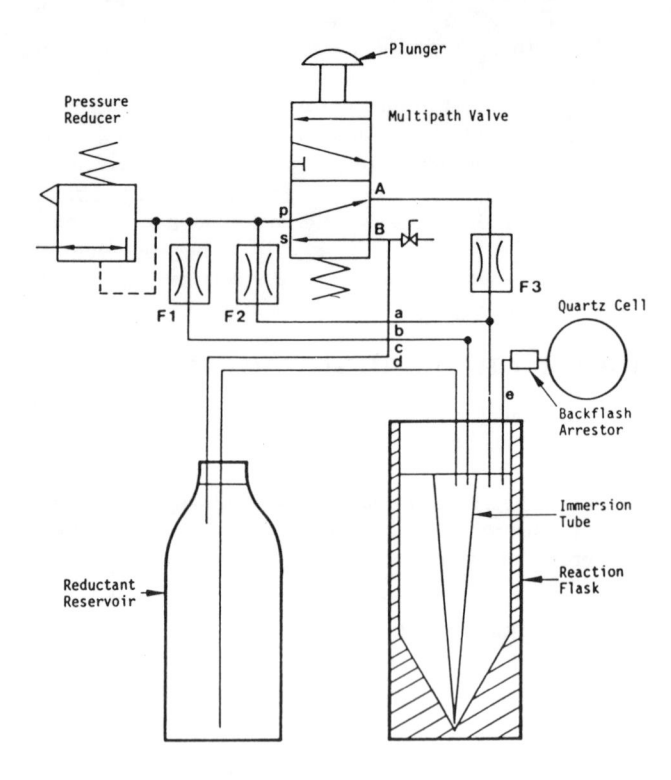

Fig. 1. Diagram of the pneumatic system of the MHS-10
Flow restrictors (F1, F2, F3), flow lines (a-e), and other labeled components discussed in text

immediately and the flow of the purge gas via F_3 is resumed. The reaction proceeds rapidly to completion, after which the reaction flask can be removed and the next sample prepared.

A pressure-relief valve fitted to outlet B opens if the pressure in the reductant reservoir exceeds 4 kPa. This safety feature prevents excessive pressure build-up in the system should the sample-transfer tube or backflash arrestor become obstructed for any reason.

Reagents and Standards

Reagents were obtained from Fisher Scientific Co., Pittsburgh, PA, but materials from other sources give equivalent results.

1. *Antifoam B* (no. A-128).
2. *Dilute nitric acid, 0.24 mol/L*. Add 7.5 mL of concentrated HNO_3 to 250 mL of de-ionized water and dilute to 500 mL. This solution is stable for a year when stored in a brown glass bottle at room temperature.
3. *Sodium borohydride, 0.79 mol/L*. Dilute 5 g of NaOH to 500 mL with de-ionized water. Add 15 g of $NaBH_4$ and filter. Refrigerated at 4-7 °C, this solution is stable for two weeks.
4. *$KMnO_4$, 0.32 mol/L*. Dissolve 5 g of solid $KMnO_4$ in 100 mL of de-ionized water. This solution is stable for a year when stored in a brown glass bottle at 4-7 °C.
5. *Stock standard*. Mercury, 1 g/L.
6. *Working standard, 1 mg/L*. Dilute 1 mL of stock standard to 1 L with de-ionized water. This solution is stable for six months when stored in a brown glass bottle at 4-7 °C.

Collection and Handling of Specimens

Acidify 24-h urine to pH 2 with nitric acid after collection.

Note: The Evaluator found acidification to be unnecessary, with loss of mercury being neither extensive nor clinically significant.

Procedure

1. Set up standards as follows: To each of three sample cups containing 10 mL of dilute HNO_3 plus two drops of antifoam, add working standard, 0, 50, or 100 µg/L, to prepare, respectively, a blank and two mercury standards.
2. Prepare samples and control as follows: In each sample cup, mix 9 mL of dilute HNO_3, two drops of antifoam, and 1 mL of sample or control material.

Note: The Evaluator uses a Repipetor to dispense approximately 0.1 mL of antifoam.

3. Add five drops of $KMnO_4$ solution to each sample just before testing.
4. Set up the mercury hydride system according to the manufacturer's instructions, with either nitrogen or argon as the carrier gas.
5. Place each cup on the holder of the instrument and adjust the recorder to display zero. Lower the recorder pen and push the "dispense" button down. When the absorbance displayed by the recorder has peaked, release the button and lift the recorder pen. Remove the sample cup and rinse the dispenser tip with de-ionized water before adding the next sample.
6. If absorbance exceeds 0.35, use 0.5 mL of sample with 9.5 mL of dilute HNO_3 (plus antifoam) and multiply results by 2.

Quality Control

Several manufacturers, including both Fisher Scientific and Ortho Diagnostics, produce urine controls containing a concentration of mercury similar to that expected in industrial exposure.

Calculations

Measure each peak height (H), and subtract from each the peak height of the blank. Calculate the concentration of mercury from the corrected height as follows:

H unknown × concn of standard = concn of unknown, µg/L.

Results and Discussion

Data for the standard curve are presented in Table 1. Precision and recovery studies are summarized in Tables 2 and 3.

In routine use the method is rapid and offers accuracy and precision at least equal to those of other methods (3). Although urine represents a complex matrix differing widely in composition, the method of standard additions was not necessary. The analytical curve from aqueous standards has the same slope as one produced by standard additions to a urine sample (1).

Table 1. Data for Constructing Standard Curve

Mercury concn, µg/L	Absorbance readings (duplicates)
0	0.03, 0.03
10	0.045, 0.047
50	0.112, 0.110
100	0.180, 0.182
250	0.335, 0.330

Table 2. Precision Studies

	Control value, µg/L	Mercury concn, µg/L Measured	SD	CV, %
Within day				
Evaluator	193[a]	190	10.7	5.6
Submitter	101[b]	103	6.1	5.9
Day to day				
Evaluator	193[a]	187	13.8	7.4
Submitter	101[b]	105	7.8	7.4

[a]Commercial urine control from Fisher Scientific, Orangeburg, NY.
[b]Commercial urine control from Ortho Diagnostic Systems, Raritan, NJ.
n = 20 each.

Table 3. Analytical Recovery Studies

	Mercury, µg/L	Mean recovery (and range), %
Evaluator	5 - 600	97 (87 - 109)
Submitter	10 - 500	96 (90 - 105)

The method is specific for mercury although it is not selective for either organic or inorganic mercury. Both forms are reduced to elemental mercury by this method. Either the dilute nitric acid or the sodium borohydride solution may be contaminated with mercury, which will be reflected in a high absorbance reading from the blank.

Healthy individuals should have urinary mercury values of <10 µg/L (or <20 µg/24 h). In persons subject to industrial exposure, concentrations may reach 150 µg/L (5).

References

1. Analytical methods using the MHS-10 mercury/hydride system. Perkin-Elmer Corp., Norwalk, CT, October, 1978.
2. Sharma DC, Davis PC. Direct determination of mercury in blood by use of sodium borohydride reduction and atomic absorption spectrophotometry. *Clin Chem* **25**, 769-772 (1979).
3. Clarkson TW, Greenwood MR, Magos L. Atomic absorption determination of total, inorganic, and organic mercury in biological fluids. *Clinical Chemistry and Chemical Toxicology of Metals*, SS Brown, Ed., Elsevier, New York, NY, 1977, pp 201-208.
4. Aitio A, Jarvisalo J. Biological monitoring of occupational exposure to toxic chemicals. *Ann Clin Lab Sci* **15**, 121-139 (1985).
5. Clarkson TW. Mercury poisoning. *Op. cit.* (ref. 3), pp 189-200.

Methaqualone by Spectrophotometry

Submitter: Larry A. Broussard, *Medical Laboratory Associates, Birmingham, AL 35256*

Evaluators: Richard T. Tulley, *Earl K. Long Memorial Hospital, Baton Rouge, LA 70805*
C. Andrew Robinson, Jr., and Catherine H. Ketchum, *Department of Pathology, University of Alabama in Birmingham, Birmingham, AL 35294*

Introduction

Methaqualone, 2-methyl-3-*o*-tolyl-4(3*H*)-quinazolinone, is a sedative and hypnotic agent originally developed as a "safe" alternative to the barbiturates. Introduced in the United States in 1965, methaqualone was classified as a controlled drug in 1973 after reports of widespread abuse, dependency, serious overdose reactions, and severe withdrawal syndromes. After subsiding in the middle 1970s, methaqualone abuse appeared again in the late 1970s and early 1980s as counterfeit methaqualone tablets became available. In November 1983, the only domestic manufacturer of the drug (Quaalude®), Lemmon Pharmacal Co., stopped producing methaqualone. One would expect that the demand for laboratory testing of the drug would diminish, but as long as methaqualone is available illegally and is still abused, the need for monitoring it remains.

Methods available for the detection of methaqualone include thin-layer chromatography (*1-3*), gas-liquid chromatography (*4*), gas chromatography-mass spectrometry (*5,6*), radioimmunoassay (*7,8*), enzyme immunoassay (*9*), and ultraviolet spectrometry. The method presented here is the ultraviolet spectrophotometric method of Bailey and Jatlow (*10*), a quantitative method that may be modified and included in a general screen for sedative drugs (*11*).

Principle

Methaqualone is extracted into hexane from serum or gastric contents at an alkaline pH, then re-extracted into HCl, 1 mol/L. The absorbance of the HCl solution is scanned from 260 nm to 212 nm, and methaqualone is identified by its characteristic absorption spectrum. The methaqualone concentration, which is proportional to the absorbance at 235 nm, is calculated by comparison with the absorbance of an aqueous standard taken through the procedure.

Materials and Methods

Reagents

1. *Hexane:* Reagent grade may be used.

   Note: In the original procedure redistilled hexane was utilized, but this has not been necessary in the Submitter's laboratory.

2. *NaOH, 1 mol/L:* Dissolve 40 g of NaOH in water in a 1-L volumetric flask. Cool and dilute to volume with water. Stable for six months when stored at room temperature in a brown glass bottle.

3. *NaOH, 567 mmol/L:* Dissolve 22.68 g of NaOH in about 500 mL of water in a 1-L volumetric flask. Cool and dilute to volume with water. Stable for six months when stored at room temperature in a brown glass bottle.

4. *HCl, 1 mol/L:* Add 83 mL of concentrated HCl to water in a 1-L volumetric flask. Dilute to volume with water. Stable for one year when stored at room temperature in a brown glass bottle.

5. *Methaqualone stock standard, 100 mg/L:* Dissolve 10.0 mg of methaqualone (Arnar-Stone Laboratories, Inc., Mount Prospect, IL) in about 2 mL of ethanol in a 100-mL volumetric flask and dilute to volume with water. Stable for two months when stored at 2-6 °C in a brown glass bottle.

6. *Methaqualone working standard, 5 mg/L:* Dilute 5.0 mL of stock standard to volume with water in a 100-mL volumetric flask. Stable for two months when stored at 2-6 °C in a brown glass bottle.

   Note: All reagents should be stored in glass bottles. The plastic from which many bottles and tubes are manufactured contains a substance that is leached into the reagents and absorbs strongly in the ultraviolet region.

Apparatus

A recording ultraviolet spectrophotometer is required. The instrument in the Submitter's laboratory is a double-beam recording ultraviolet-visible spectrophotometer (Model 25; Beckman Instruments, Inc., Fullerton, CA). Silica cuvets of 2.5-mL capacity and 1-cm pathlength were used.

Specimens

Serum is the specimen of choice. Urine is a poor specimen for detecting methaqualone because the drug is extensively metabolized to at least five major monohydroxylated metabolites, which are excreted in the urine as glucuronide conjugates; very little, if any, unmetabolized methaqualone is excreted in the urine (*12*). Techniques for screening urine samples must be capable of detecting these metabolites. The method may be used for qualitative detection of methaqualone in gastric contents.

Procedure

1. Place 1.0 mL of water in a 16 × 125-mm screw-top tube or a 15-mL glass-stoppered centrifuge tube (blank).

   Note: Evaluators C. A. R. and C. H. K. suggest using drug-free serum as the blank to avoid the high background absorbance they observed. This phenomenon may depend on the grade of hexane or other reagents used.

2. Place 1.0 mL of working standard in a 16 × 125-mm screw-top tube or a 15-mL glass-stoppered centrifuge tube (standard).

3. Place 1.0 mL of control, serum, or gastric contents in a 16 × 125-mm screw-top tube or a 15-mL glass-stoppered centrifuge tube (control or unknown).

4. Add 0.10 mL of 1 mol/L NaOH to each tube and mix.

5. Add 10.0 mL of hexane to each tube. (A calibrated dispenser is helpful.)

6. Shake the contents of each tube on a mechanical shaker for 5 min.

> *Note:* Evaluator R. T. T. reports that an automatic rocker-type blood mixer may be utilized. In this case the time of shaking in step 6 should be increased to 15 min, and the times in steps 9 and 12 increased to 5 min.

7. Allow the layers to separate (centrifuge if necessary) and transfer 8.0 mL of the hexane (upper) layer to a 16 × 125-mm screw-top tube or a 15-mL glass-stoppered centrifuge tube.

8. Add 3.0 mL of 567 mmol/L NaOH to each tube.

9. Shake each tube on a mechanical shaker for 1 min.

10. Allow the layers to separate and transfer 6.0 mL of the hexane (upper) layer to another 16 × 125-mm screw-top tube or 15-mL glass-stoppered centrifuge tube.

11. Add 3.0 mL of 1 mol/L HCl to each tube.

12. Shake each tube on a mechanical shaker for 1 min.

13. Allow the layers to separate, then aspirate and discard the hexane (upper) layer.

14. Transfer the HCl layer to a 1-cm cuvet and record the absorbances of the standard, control, and unknowns from 260 nm to 212 nm against the blank. At the beginning of each scan (260 nm) it may be necessary to adjust the pen to zero absorbance.

> *Note:* Evaluator R. T. T. reports that when a single-beam recording spectrophotometer is used, one must adjust the instrument to zero at 260 nm for each sample and the blank. Subtract the absorbance (or peak height) at 235 nm for the blank from the absorbance (or peak height) at 235 nm for each sample and use these values in the calculation.

15. Mark the absorbance at 235 nm. Draw the baseline for each specimen parallel to the x-axis of the graph, using the initial portion of the curve as a guide. Measure the peak height and (or) absorbance at 235 nm.

Calculation

$$\frac{A_{235} \text{ unknown}}{A_{235} \text{ standard}} \times 5 = \text{methaqualone, mg/L}$$

When a spectrophotometer that reads absorbance directly and a linear recorder are used, peak heights at 235 nm may be substituted for absorbance at 235 nm in the calculation.

Results and Discussion

Interpretation

Methaqualone is a synthetic compound; the "normal" concentration, therefore, is zero. Report "none detected" for any specimen giving results of 1 mg/L or less. For gastric specimens, report as "none detected" for specimens giving no measurable absorbance at 235 nm or as "positive" if a measurable peak at 235 nm is observed.

Expected Values

Methaqualone is rapidly absorbed (99% within 2 h). The interpretation of serum concentrations depends on the methodology used. Ultraviolet spectrometric methods involving chloroform and ether extracts yield higher concentrations because metabolites are also measured (*11*). In a study in which the procedure presented here was used, Bailey (*13*) concluded that methaqualone concentrations exceeding 9 mg/L were always associated with a depressed level of consciousness but that below this value there was no significant correlation between serum concentrations and physical findings.

Analytical Variables

Linearity and sensitivity. Beer's law is followed for methaqualone concentrations up to 40 mg/L. For concentrations exceeding 40 mg/L, the sample must be diluted with water and reassayed. Methaqualone can be reproducibly detected and quantified in concentrations as low as 1 mg/L.

> *Note:* Evaluator R. T. T. reports that the method is linear to 60 mg/L and that, even at 100 mg/L, there was minimal deviation from linearity.

Analytical recovery. The recovery data for drug-free serum to which methaqualone was added (as compared with the aqueous standard taken through the procedure) are shown in Table 1. Bailey and Jatlow (*10*) reported the uncorrected recovery of methaqualone by this method to be 50-55% and recommended the use of serum standards. Based on the analytical recoveries shown in Table 1, it does not appear to be necessary to use serum standards, as long as the aqueous standard is taken through the entire procedure.

Table 1. Analytical Recovery Studies

	Methaqualone, mg/L	n	Mean recovery (and range), %
Evaluator R. T. T.	5	2	94 (89-100)
	10	2	98 (97-100)
	20	2	99 (98-101)
	30	2	105 (104-106)
	40	2	107 (103-112)
Evaluators C.A.R. and C.H.K.	2	20	108 (70-165)
	5	20	99 (79-131)
	10	20	100 (88-110)
	40	20	96 (91-106)
Submitter	2	2	100 (98-102)
	5	2	102 (98-106)
	10	2	100 (96-104)
	20	2	93 (91- 95)
	40	2	98 (94-104)

Precision. The precision data obtained by the analysis of a pooled specimen are shown in Table 2.

Specificity. For a drug to interfere with this method it would have to: reach measurable concentrations in serum, be extracted by the procedure, and absorb strongly in the ultraviolet region. The alkaloids, amphetamines, tricyclic antidepressants, and phenothiazines do not reach concentrations in serum high enough to cause interference. Barbiturates are sparingly soluble in hexane and would be removed by the NaOH wash. Chlordiazepoxide does not interfere at a concentration of 2 mg/L. Diazepam and antihistamines will yield characteristic spectra that prevent the quantification of methaqualone (10), but that also call attention to the presence an interfering compound, thereby avoiding the possibility of the report of a falsely increased concentration of methaqualone.

Table 2. Precision Studies

Methaqualone concn, mg/L			
Mean	SD	n	CV, %
Within-run precision			
10.2	0.42	20	4.2
4.8	0.21	20	4.3
Run-to-run precision			
2.2	0.60	20	24.9
5.0	0.70	20	14.0
10.0	0.70	20	7.0
7.0[a]	0.97[a]	43[a]	13.8[a]

[a] Day-to-day precision obtained from the routine analysis of a pooled specimen by at least six technologists in the Submitter's laboratory. Other results are from Evaluators C. A. R. and C. H. K.

References

1. Sleeman HK, Cella JA, Harvey JL, Beach DJ. Thin-layer chromatographic detection and identification of methaqualone metabolites in urine. *Clin Chem* **21**, 76-80 (1975).
2. Goudie JH, Burnett D. A rapid method for the detection of methaqualone metabolites. *Clin Chim Acta* **35**, 133-135 (1971).
3. Burnet D, Goudie JH, Sherrif JM. Detection of methaqualone and its metabolites in urine. *J Clin Pathol* **22**, 602-604 (1969).
4. Mitchard M, Williams ME. An improved quantitative gas-liquid chromatographic assay for the estimation of methaqualone in biological fluids. *J Chromatogr* **72**, 29-34 (1972).
5. Bonnichsen R, Fri CG, Negoita C, Ryhage R. Identification of methaqualone metabolites from urine extracted by gas chromatography-mass spectrometry. *Clin Chim Acta* **40**, 309-318 (1972).
6. Bonnichsen R, Marde Y, Ryhage R. Identification of free and conjugated metbolites of methaqualone by gas chromatography-mass spectrometry. *Clin Chem* **20**, 230-235 (1974).
7. Berman AR, McGrath JP, Permisohn RC, Cella JA. Radioimmunoassay of methaqualone and its monohydroxy metabolites in urine. *Clin Chem* **21**, 1878-1881 (1975).
8. Bost RO, Sutheimer CA, Sunshine I. Methaqualone assay by radioimmunoassay and gas chromatography. *Clin Chem* **22**, 689-690 (1976).
9. Oellerich M. Enzyme immunoassays in clinical chemistry: Present status and trends. *J Clin Chem Clin Biochem* **18**, 197-208 (1980).
10. Bailey DN, Jatlow PI. Methaqualone overdose: Analytical methodology and the significance of serum drug concentrations. *Clin Chem* **19**, 615-620 (1973).
11. Jatlow PI. *Methodology for Analytical Toxicology*, CRC Press, Inc., Cleveland, OH, 1975, pp 414-420.
12. Kazyak L, Kelley JA, Cella JA, et al. Methaqualone metabolites in human urine after therapeutic doses. *Clin Chem* **23**, 2001-2006 (1977).
13. Bailey DV. Methaqualone ingestion: Evaluation of present status. *J Anal Toxicol* **5**, 279-282 (1981).

Osmolality of Serum for Evaluating the Acutely Intoxicated Patient

Submitters: Alexandros A. Pappas and Richard H. Gadsden, Sr., *Department of Laboratory Medicine, Medical University of South Carolina, Charleston, SC 29425*

Evaluators: William H. Porter, *Department of Pathology, University of Kentucky Medical Center, Lexington, KY 40536*
Richard E. Mullins, *Department of Pathology, Laboratory Medicine, Emory University, Atlanta, GA 30322*

Introduction

Emergency determinations of blood alcohol (ethanol) are frequently requested of clinical laboratories. The methods used for this depend on the available equipment and technologist expertise (1). The indirect detection of alcohols, through their measurable and predictable effect on serum osomolality (2), is rapid and simple and preserves the sample for additional analyses when only minimal sample volume is available (3).

Ethanol (EtOH) is the most frequently encountered alcohol in acutely intoxicated individuals and is the most common extrinsic cause of increased serum osmolality (4). The presence of nonvolatile drugs does not significantly affect the serum osmolality. The concentration of EtOH can be estimated by subtracting the calculated serum osmolality (C-Osm) from the measured serum osmolality (M-Osm), to obtain the "delta-osmolality": Δ-Osm (5). This estimation may not differentiate between EtOH and significant amounts of other volatiles (e.g., methanol, isopropanol, ethylene glycol, acetone), nor is it sensitive enough for use in forensic cases; however, the specificity and sensitivity of the results obtained can be improved for clinical cases by the rapid determination of serum EtOH enzymatically with alcohol dehydrogenase (see pp. 63-65). In addition, gas chromatography (see pp. 40-43) can be used if the amount of enzymatically determined EtOH (if present) does not account for the observed Δ-Osm.

Principle

When a solute is dissolved in a solvent, four of the properties of the solvent are changed so as to vary linearly with the amount of solute added: (a) the freezing point is lowered; (b) the boiling point is raised; (c) the osmotic pressure is increased; and (d) the vapor pressure is lowered. These colligative properties change with solute concentration—not in proportion to the molecular mass, size, or shape of the solute particles, but only according to the number of solute particles involved. The osmolality of serum is primarily (92%) the result of effects of sodium (Na^+), chloride (Cl^-), and bicarbonate (HCO_3^-), the remaining 8% being accounted for by the other serum electrolytes, proteins, glucose, and urea nitrogen.

Although serum osmolality is commonly measured by freezing-point or vapor pressure (dew-point) depression, the vapor pressure osmometer will not respond to a free volatile solute, such as EtOH, because the total vapor pressure consists of both solvent and solute vapor pressure. To assess the presence and estimate the concentration of serum EtOH, one must therefore measure serum osmolality by freezing-point depression (6).

There are several formulae for calculating serum osmolality (7). A commonly used and accurate formula, presented by Glasser et al. (5), is:

$$\text{mOsm/kg } H_2O = \frac{1.86\, Na + \dfrac{\text{glucose}}{180} + \dfrac{\text{urea-N}}{28}}{0.93} \quad (1)$$

where Na is in mmol/L, glucose in mg/L, and urea-N in mg/L

1.86 = constant for the electro-osmotic coefficient and dissociation constant for sodium chloride
180 = conversion of glucose from mg/L to mmol/L
28 = conversion of urea-N from mg/L to mmol/L
0.93 = corrects for the percentage of serum water.

This reduces conveniently to:

$$\text{mOsm/kg } H_2O = 2\, Na + 0.005\, \text{glucose} + 0.036\, \text{urea-N} \quad (2)$$

The presence of EtOH in serum depresses the freezing point of serum, which results in a linearly related increase of the M-Osm. The observable difference between the M-Osm and C-Osm can thus be used to estimate the quantity of EtOH in the serum (Figure 1). Figure 2 demonstrates the effects of other common volatile materials on Δ-Osm in serum.

Concentrations of the various serum volatiles can be estimated from the Δ-Osm value by using the respective relative molecular masses to obtain conversion factors (Table 1).

Table 1. Relative Molecular Masses (M_r) of Volatile Compounds and Effect (at 1000 mg/L) on Serum Δ-Osm Determined by Freezing-Point Depression

Compound	M_r	Δ-Osm[a]
Methanol	32	31.3
Ethanol	46	21.7
Isopropanol	60	16.7
Ethylene glycol	62	16.1
Acetone	58	17.2

[a] mOsm/kg H_2O.

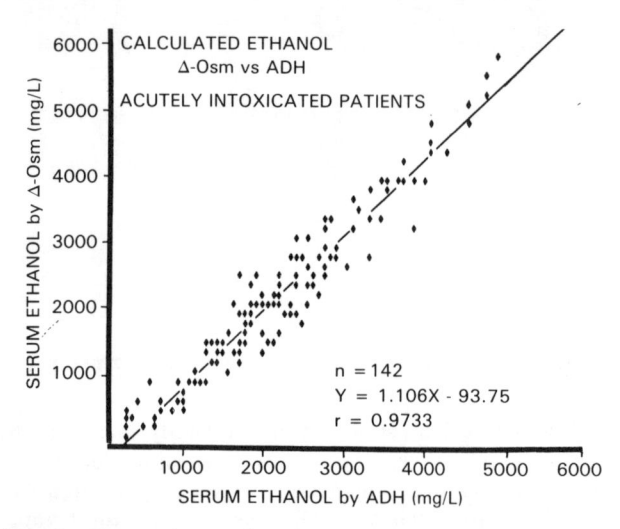

Fig. 1. Comparison of estimated serum ethanol Δ-Osm values with enzymically determined ethanol in 142 clinical cases

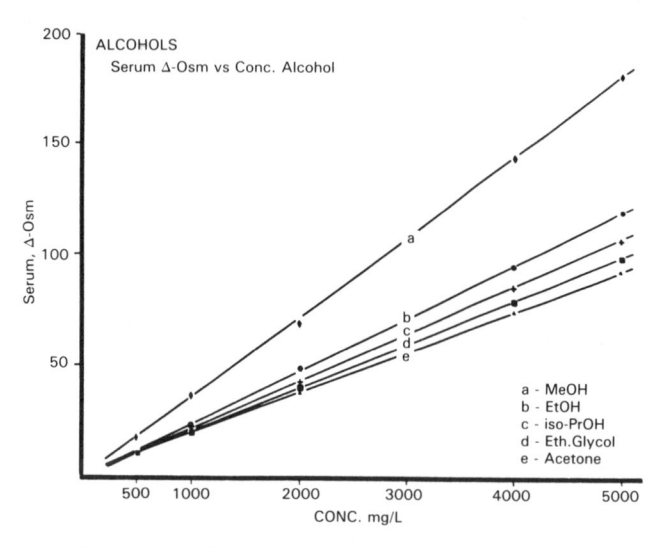

Fig. 2. Effects of low-M_r alcohols (from top to bottom: methanol, ethanol, isopropanol, ethylene glycol, and acetone) on Δ-Osm values

Evaluator R.E.M. found the ΔOsm method accurately predicted the concentration of EtOH, methanol (MeOH), and acetone. The equations and correlations are as follows:
EtOH (mg/dL) = 3.88 (Δ-Osm) − 28.9; r = 0.998
MeOH (mg/dL) = 3.88 (Δ-Osm) − 27.0; r = 0.996
Acetone (mg/dL) = 8.75 (Δ-Osm) − 93.5; r = 0.986

Materials and Methods

Reagents

Osmolality standards, 100 and 500 mOsm/kg of H_2O. Weigh 0.30 g and 1.5717 g of NaCl (certified ACS, cat. no. 271; Fisher Scientific Co., Pittsburgh, PA 15238) and dissolve each in 100 g of distilled water. The osmolalities are 100 and 500 mOsm/kg of H_2O, respectively.

Commercial freezing-point osmometry standards are available, from Advanced Instruments, Inc., Needham Heights, MA 02194 (100 mOsm/kg, cat. no. 3LA010; 500 mOsm/kg, cat. no. 3LA050) and Precision Instruments, Inc., Sudbury, MA 01776 (100 mOsm/kg, stock no. 2101; 500 mOsm/kg, stock no. 2105). We have found these standards to be accurate in comparison with in-house-prepared osmolality standards.

Apparatus

The choice of osmometer is left to the user but must be cryoscopic (based on freezing-point depression) in principle. We have found the following instruments to be reliable, accurate, and amenable to rapid throughput: Advanced Digimatic Osmometer (Model 3DII; Advanced Instruments) and Osmette A (Model 500-2; Precision Instruments, Inc.).

The respective manufacturer's specifications suffice for determining serum osmolality. To check the instrument's calibration, choose standards that bracket the expected serum osmolality (reference range for M-Osm = 277 to 297 mOsm/kg). We recommend calibrating at least once a day.

The accuracy of these instruments is within 1.0 mOsm/kg of the "all methods" mean established by the College of American Pathologists' survey program, within a CV of <2.0% (8).

Collection and Handling of Specimens

Collect an adequate number of samples from acutely intoxicated patients, to be used for the rapid initial patient evaluation and for follow-up, as indicated.

a. Collect at least 14 mL of clotted blood into two 7-mL sterile, evacuated tubes without additive (no. 4736, Becton Dickinson Co., Rutherford, NJ 07070; or equivalent). These specimens are used to prepare serum samples for measuring osmolality and the concentrations of Na, glucose, urea-N, and EtOH. Allow to clot for 30 min, then centrifuge at 3000 × g for 5 min at room temperature with stoppers in place (to avoid loss of any volatile material). Analyze without delay.

Cover the remaining serum sample with Parafilm and store at 4 °C for definitive drug assays if indicated.

b. Collect at least 14 mL of anticoagulated blood into two 7-mL sterile, evacuated tubes containing EDTA (no. 6450, Becton Dickinson Co., or equivalent). This whole-blood sample is used for follow-up analysis of volatile materials other than or in addition to EtOH, if indicated. Gas chromatography for common volatiles, such as methanol and isopropanol (9) or plasma ethylene glycol (10), is the method of choice if more specific results are needed relatively quickly.

c. Collect at least 30 mL of urine for additional assessment of drug presence, if indicated. Thin-layer chromatography and gas chromatography are convenient and rapid methods for qualitative drug analysis.

Procedures

1. Determine the M-Osm of the patient's sample by freezing-point osmometry.
2. Measure serum glucose emzymically, by the hexokinase (11) or glucose oxidase (12) methods.
3. Measure urea-N in serum, enzymically by the urease-rate method (13) or with ion-selective electrodes (14).
4. Measure serum Na by flame photometry (15) or with ion-selective electrodes (16).
5. Calculate C-Osm from equation 1 or 2.
6. Calculate the Δ-Osm by subtracting C-Osm from M-Osm.

For verification of the EtOH content in serum, we have found that the following enzymic commercial kits are convenient and yield identical results:

1. Alcohol (ALC) single pack for the *aca* (Du Pont Chemical Systems Div., Wilmington, DE 19898).
2. Single-assay vial NAD-ADH (Sigma Chemical Co.,

stock no. 301-1), and multiple-assay vial (stock no. 332-5). These have been optimized for linearity up to 3000 mg/L (17).

3. Multiple-assay vial, "Alcohol Stat-Pak" (Calbiochem, Summerville, NJ 00876; cat. no. 869-219).

4. Alcohol multiple assay kit (Boehringer-Mannheim Diagnostics, Indianapolis, IN 46520; stock no. 123960).

Calculations

The Δ-Osm should be essentially zero (± 10) if no EtOH or other low-M_r volatile is present in the sample. For each 1000 mg of EtOH per liter of serum, the Δ-Osm will increase by 21.7 mOsm/kg. The estimation of EtOH from Δ-Osm and the concordance with the enzymically determined EtOH values are shown in Figure 3. The computation of the C-Osm and Δ-Osm for automatic comparison with serum EtOH, to detect significant discrepancies (>10 mOsm/kg), may be programmed on a calculator or microcomputer (3).

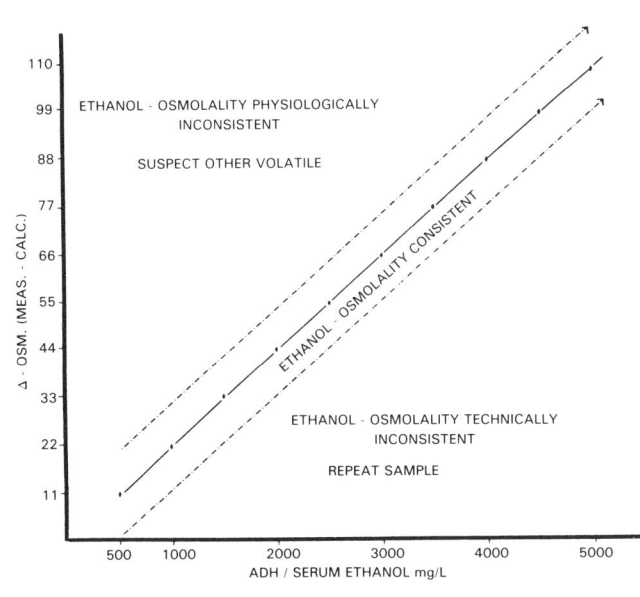

Fig. 3. A comparison of concentrations of ethanol in serum with Δ-Osm values, indicating the areas of discrepancy that require laboratory action

Quality Control

Quality-control (QC) material for determining osmolality should have a protein base. We have found commercially available routine chemistry controls satisfactory for this purpose because of stability and lot number longevity. Including a single QC serum sample with each patient's sample is adequate. There is no Δ-Osm QC material available commercially. Moreover, in-house preparations are unsatisfactory primarily because of the volatile nature of the analyte (EtOH).

A negative Δ-Osm (C-Osm > M-Osm) is usually indicative of an error in: (*a*) the calculation of Δ-Osm or C-Osm; or (*b*) the analysis of serum M-Osm, glucose, urea-N, or, in particular, Na$^+$.

A Δ-Osm > 20 mOsm/kg, in the absence of low-M_r volatiles or other presumed but unmeasured anions, may indicate contamination of the sample by some osmotically active extrinsic material, i.e., EDTA, fluoride, oxalate, etc.

Evaluator R.E.M. reported run-to-run precision (CV) for Δ-Osm as 6% at an EtOH concentration of 1 g/L and 3% at an EtOH concentration of 2.5 g/L (n = 30 each).

Results and Discussion

The mean (± SD) M-Osm in 55 healthy young adults was 285.1 (± 4.3) mOsm/kg; the C-Osm for these sera was 290.0 (± 5.1) mOsm/kg. The respective reference intervals for these values were 277-297 and 278-299 mOsm/kg. The CV was less than 2.0%.

The patient's C-Osm value serves as its own reference value. A Δ-Osm increase of less than 10 mOsm/kg may rapidly rule out the presence of clinically significant concentrations of low-M_r volatiles and, in particular, EtOH. An increased Δ-Osm value (>10 mOsm/kg) due to EtOH can be readily verified by an enzymic determination of serum EtOH and thus rule out the presence of any significant amounts of other low-M_r volatiles except probably ethylene glycol. Significant discrepancies (Δ-Osm > 10 mOsm/kg) between concentrations of serum EtOH determined osmotically and enzymically must be resolved (3, 19).

Determination of the M-Osm, C-Osm, Δ-Osm, and major serum constituents may lead to rapid evaluation of metabolic causes of altered mental status if alcohol or drug intoxication is not indicated. Metabolic disorders such as hyperglycemia, uremia, or dehydration will increase both the measured and the calculated osmolality (18). Intrinsic metabolic conditions do not usually significantly increase the Δ-Osm.

The presence of unmeasured analytes such as lactate and acetone, which may be present in such metabolic derangements, are readily apparent from the clinical appearance and initial laboratory data, e.g., pH, anion gap, glucose, and serum acetone. The Δ-Osm discrepancy, if any, in such cases is usually in the range of 10 to 15 mOsm/kg.

When there are no apparent intrinsic metabolic causes for a Δ-Osm/enzymic EtOH discrepancy, further differentiation between EtOH and an ingested unknown alcohol may be suggested from additional laboratory determinations (Table 2).

One can estimate the effect of the suspected volatile by using the relative molecular mass of the respective volatile (Table 1) and the following equation:

Concentration, g/L = Δ-Osm × M_r

If the estimate does not appear reasonable, one can then quickly decide whether to verify the presence of the suspected volatile with a definitive analytical procedure, such as gas chromatography.

In conclusion, the serum values for Δ-Osm can rapidly and simply rule out clinically significant quantities of low-M_r volatile toxic materials. Comparison of the serum Δ-Osm with the enzymically measured serum EtOH is a rapid, simple, and independent method for detecting low-

Table 2. Characteristic Laboratory Findings Associated with Commonly Ingested Alcohols

Alcohol	Δ-Osm	pH	Anion gap	Serum acetone	Urinary oxalate
Ethanol	↑	NC[a]	NC[a]	NC[a]	NC
Methanol	↑	↓	↑	NC	NC
Isopropanol	↑	NC	NC	↑	NC
Ethylene glycol	↑	↓	↑	NC	↑

NC = No significant change.
[a] Not decreased or present unless alcoholic ketoacidosis supervenes.

M_r volatile compounds commonly found in acutely intoxicated patients.

Evaluator R.E.M.'s Comments

The method is useful to rapidly estimate and confirm serum concentrations of EtOH in intoxicated patients. It is probably more useful as a method to rule out methanol, isopropanol, acetone, or other volatiles as possible intoxicants when the increase in Δ-Osm is < 10 mOsm/kg and no EtOH is found by enzymic assay for EtOH.

Evaluator W.H.P.'s Comments

Correlation studies with patients' samples. Thirty separate patients' serum specimens submitted to the clinical toxicology laboratory for analysis of volatiles (acetone, isopropanol, methanol, and EtOH) by head-space gas chromatography were also analyzed for osmolality (Advanced Instruments freezing-point depression osmometer) and for serum Na, glucose, and urea-N (Beckman Astra). The calculated Δ-Osm was plotted against the measured EtOH concentration. All but two of the patients' results fell within the reference interval relating EtOH concentration to Δ-Osm. One of the patients whose Δ-Osm was greater than the expected range had received mannitol intravenously en route to the emergency room; the other patient had volatile substances present in addition to EtOH (EtOH, 2360 mg/L; isopropanol, 160 mg/L; acetone, 300 mg/L). Thus, in each case, the relationship of Δ-Osm to serum EtOH accurately indicated the presence of osmotically active solutes other than EtOH.

The EtOH concentration for each specimen was also calculated from the Δ-Osm, on the assumption that EtOH was the only osmotically active constituent responsible for the increased Δ-Osm. This calculated EtOH concentration was then plotted against the measured EtOH concentration, omitting the two specimens known to contain osmotically active constituents in addition to EtOH. The regression equation relating the calculated EtOH (y) to the measured EtOH (x) was $y = 1.03x + 6.5$ mg/dL ($r = 0.9917$, n = 28).

Precision: Precision studies for Δ-Osm calculations were not performed. Each of the analytical procedures involved in this calculation, however, is subjected to routine quality-control measures.

Discussion: The relationship of Δ-Osm to serum EtOH concentration appears to be valuable in evaluating the acutely intoxicated patient, especially for laboratories that do not have the facilities to identify and quantify on an emergency basis the specific alcohols or ethylene glycol. However, the potential limitation of this approach with regard to sensitivity for detecting the presence of ethylene glycol, acetone, and other alcohols should be clearly recognized, and may be especially important in cases of ethylene glycol intoxication. For instance, an ethylene glycol concentration of 500 mg/L in serum would theoretically result in a Δ-Osm of about 8, within the range of normal variation of the Δ-Osm determination (≤10). Serum concentrations of ethylene glycol as low as 300 mg/L have been observed in cases of fatal ethylene glycol intoxication (*20*). Moreover, the half-life of ethylene glycol is about 3 h (*21*), and its concentration in serum may therefore decline relatively rapidly. If there is a significant delay (6-8 h) between the time of peak absorption and blood sampling, ethylene glycol may be measured as 500 mg/L in severe cases of intoxication, in which the peak serum concentration may have been in the range of 2000 mg/L. Nevertheless, it would be important to establish ethylene glycol as the causative toxic agent. Similar concerns apply to the detection of methanol, concentrations as low as 230-300 mg/L having been observed in serious or fatal cases (*22,23*). The anticipated Δ-Osm at this concentration range would be approximately 7-9, again perhaps within the normal deviation of the measurements.

Laboratories that utilize this method should exercise caution in evaluating a normal Δ-Osm value for a patient with a history and presentation suggestive of consumption of ethylene glycol, isopropanol, or methanol.

References

1. Dubowski KM. Alcohol determination in the clinical laboratory. *Am J Clin Pathol* **74**, 747-750 (1980).
2. Redetzki HM, Koerner TA, Hughes JR, Smith AG. Osmometry in the evaluation of alcohol intoxication. *Clin Toxicol* **5**, 343-363 (1972).
3. Pappas AA, Gadsden RH Jr, Gadsden RH Sr, Groves WE. Computerized calculation of osmolality and its automatic comparison with observed serum ethanol concentration. *Am J Clin Pathol* **77**, 449-451 (1982).
4. Robinson AG, Loeb JN. Ethanol ingestion—commonest cause of elevated plasma osmolality? *N Engl J Med* **284**, 1253-1255 (1971).
5. Glasser L, Sternglanz PD, Combie J, Robinson A. Serum osmolality and its application to drug overdose. *Am J Clin Pathol* **60**, 695-699 (1973).
6. Barlow WK. Volatiles and osmometry. *Clin Chem* **22**, 1230-1233 (1976).
7. Dorwart WV, Chalmers L. Comparison of methods for calculating serum osmolality from chemical concentrations, and the prognostic value of such calculations. *Clin Chem* **21**, 190-194 (1973).
8. Juel R. Serum osmolality, CAP survey analysis. *Am J Clin Pathol* **68**, *Suppl*, 102-105 (1984).
9. Gadsden RH, Taylor EH. Measurements of alcohol in biological fluids. In *Manual of Procedures for the Seminar on the Clinical Pathology of Liver and Biliary Tract*, FW Sunderman, Ed., Institute for Clinical Sciences, Inc., Philadelphia, PA 19103, 1983, pp 145-152.
10. Porter WH, Anasakul A. Gas chromatographic determination of ethylene glycol in serum. *Clin Chem* **28**, 75-78 (1982).
11. Neeley WE. Simple automated determination of serum or plasma glucose by hexokinase/glucose-6-phosphate dehydrogenase method. *Clin Chem* **18**, 509-515 (1982).
12. Kadish AHB, Little RL, Sternberry JC. A new and rapid method for the determination of glucose by measurement of rate of oxygen consumption. *Clin Chem* **14**, 116-131 (1968).
13. Horak E, Sunderman FW, Sunderman FW Jr. Measurement of serum urea nitrogen by conductivimetric urease assay. *Ann Clin Lab Sci* **2**, 425-431 (1972).
14. Hanson DJ, Bretz NS. Evaluation of a semi-automated blood urea nitrogen analyzer. *Clin Chem* **23**, 477-484 (1977).
15. Boling EA. A flame photometer with simultaneous digital readout for sodium and potassium. *J Lab Clin Med* **63**, 501-510 (1964).
16. Ion-selective electrode. aca manual, Du Pont Instruments, Wilmington, DE, p 7.
17. Taylor EH, Pappas AA, Gadsden RH. Extended linearity of the Sigma alcohol procedure. *Clin Chem* **30**, 334 (1984). Letter.
18. Gennari JF. Serum osmolality, current concepts. *N Engl J Med* **310**, 102-105 (1984).
19. Vasiliades J, Pollack J, Robinson CA. Pitfalls of the alcohol dehydrogenase procedure for the emergency assay of alcohol. A case study of isopropyl overdose. *Clin Chem* **24**, 383-385 (1978).
20. Baselt RC. *Disposition of Toxic Drugs and Chemicals in Man*, 2nd ed., Biomedical Publications, Davis, CA, 1982, p 318.
21. Peterson CD, et al. Ethylene glycol poisoning. *N Engl J Med* **304**, 21-23 (1981).
22. Kane RL, et al. A methanol poisoning outbreak in Kentucky. *Arch Environ Health* **17**, 119-129 (1968).
23. Tonkabony SEH. Post-mortem blood concentration of methanol in 17 cases of fatal poisoning from contraband vodka. *Forens Sci* **6**, 1-3 (1975).

Salicylate by Spectrophotometry

Submitters: Donald E. Sutherland and John A. Lott, *Department of Pathology, The Ohio State University, Columbus, OH 43210*

Evaluator: Stan Marenberg, *Kettering Medical Center, Kettering, OH 45459*

Introduction

Acetylsalicylic acid (aspirin) and its derivatives are the most widely used drugs in the world. Aspirin is a unique drug, having analgesic, antipyretic, and anti-inflammatory properties (1). It inhibits platelet aggregation (2), probably by the acetylation of platelet proteins (3). Owing to its antiplatelet effect, it may decrease the incidence of acute myocardial infarction (4). Aspirin in large doses (more than 5 g per day) has a uricosuric effect; in doses of less than 2 g per day, it decreases urinary uric acid elimination (1). The therapeutic serum concentrations of salicylate are 20 to 100 mg/L as an analgesic-antipyretic, and 100 to 250 mg/L as an anti-inflammatory agent (1).

The three principal pathways of salicylate metabolism are the formation of salicyluric acid, salicylphenolic glucuronide, and gentisic acid. The metabolic pathways become saturated at low concentrations of salicylate, and the elimination kinetics are thus dose dependent. The metabolites are excreted rapidly, so that for practical purposes, only significant concentrations of unchanged salicylate are in the blood and tissues (5). For small doses of aspirin, e.g., 600 mg in an adult, the average half-life of the drug in blood is 2 to 3 h. With larger doses, and when anti-inflammatory concentrations in serum of about 150 mg/L are reached, the half-life is in the range of 15 to 30 h (3). Small increments in dose can lead to disproportionately large increases in serum salicylate as saturation kinetics are reached. Increasing the aspirin dose from 65 to 100 mg per kg of body weight per day triples the steady-state serum concentrations (6). Because the upper therapeutic and toxic concentrations are close together, measurements of serum salicylate are recommended for patients on prolonged high-dose aspirin therapy.

Side effects such as tinnitus and vertigo are common at serum concentrations exceeding 200 mg/L; reversible hepatotoxicity may be observed at 200-400 mg/L. Above 400 mg/L, hyperventilation producing respiratory alkalosis is common. If metabolic acidosis supervenes, the toxicity of salicylate is much greater, because more of the non-ionized form is available to penetrate the lipophilic tissues of the brain. A decrease in pH from 7.4 to 7.2 doubles the concentration of the non-ionized form and worsens the toxicity (5). The prognosis is gravest in cases with high serum concentrations of salicylate and acidemia. Methyl salicylate, e.g., as found in oil of wintergreen, is probably the most toxic of the salicylate group (3). Treatment for salicylate overdose should be directed toward producing an alkaline urine and mild metabolic alkalosis.

The severity of the toxic effect and outcome depend on the amount of salicylate ingested, and the time interval between ingestion and measurement. If the time of ingestion is known, the theoretical salicylate concentration at time zero can be estimated with the formula:

$$\log S_0 = \log S + 0.015\,T$$

where S is the salicylate concentration in the hours (T) since ingestion, and S_0 is the concentration at time zero (7). A nomogram of this equation is also available (7). S_0 concentrations have been associated with the severity of salicylate intoxication as follows (7): less than 500 mg/L, not intoxicated; 500 to 800 mg/L, mild intoxication; 800 to 1000 mg/L, moderate intoxication; above 1000 mg/L, severe intoxication; above 1600 mg/L, usually fatal. S_0 concentrations of 1600 mg/L or greater appear to be incompatible with life unless measures such as hemodialysis or exchange transfusions are used (5).

We describe a modification of the Trinder method for determining salicylate (8), and use only 0.1 mL of specimen. The Trinder method is widely used because of its simplicity, combining protein precipitation and color formation in a single step. Similar colorimetric methods are described elsewhere (9).

Principle

The Trinder method is based on the formation of color when salicylate reacts with ferric ion in an acidic medium. The purple chromophore (structure unknown) absorbs at 540 nm. The reaction is not specific; the reagent also reacts with salicylate derivatives, which ordinarily are present in inconsequential concentrations. Mercuric chloride in the acidic medium precipitates the serum proteins, thus obviating the need for a serum blank.

Materials and Methods

Reagents

Use analytical reagent-grade chemicals and distilled water throughout.

1. *Trinder's reagent*: $HgCl_2$ 80 mmol/L, $Fe(NO_3)_3$ 100 mmol/L, HCl 120 mmol/L. Dissolve 40 g of $HgCl_2$ in about 600 mL of hot water, stir to hasten dissolution, and allow the solution to cool. Add 40 g of ferric nitrate [$Fe(NO_3)_3 \cdot 9\,H_2O$] and 120 mL of 1 mol/L HCl with stirring. Transfer all the solution to a 1000-mL volumetric flask, and dilute to the mark with water. The reagent, which should be light yellow, is stable at least one year at room temperature.

2. *Stock salicylate standard, 2 g/L.* Dissolve 580 mg of sodium salicylate (HOC$_6$H$_4$COONa) in about 200 mL of water in a 250-mL volumetric flask. Add a few drops of chloroform as a preservative, and dilute to the mark with water. This solution is stable for at least five months at 4–10 °C if stored in a brown bottle.

3. *Working salicylate standard, 200 mg/L.* Dilute the stock salicylate standard 10-fold with water in a volumetric flask. Add a few drops of chloroform if the standard is to be stored. The standard is stable for at least three months when stored in a brown bottle.

4. *Controls.* Use commercially available controls. Alternatively, prepare controls by adding sodium salicylate to a serum pool as described elsewhere (9).

Instrument

Use a spectrophotometer with a bandpass of 20 nm or less set to 540 nm.

Collection and Handling of Specimens

Serum is the specimen of choice, although plasma containing EDTA, heparin, or oxalate as anticoagulants can be used. Spinal fluid and urine (9) can also be analyzed. In urine collected for 72 h after a 3-g oral dose of aspirin, only 20% of the salicylate is present in an unmetabolized form (5,10).

Analytical Procedure

1. Label 13 × 100 mm test tubes as patients' specimens or controls. Label two 12 × 75 mm cuvets as "standard" and "blank." Also label a set of 12 × 75 mm cuvets for the patients' specimens and controls.

2. Add 0.1 mL of patient's serum or control to each of the 13 × 100 mm tubes. Add 0.1 mL of standard or 0.1 mL of water to the respective standard and blank cuvets.

3. To all tubes, add 1 mL of water, mix, then add 1 mL of Trinder reagent and vortex-mix thoroughly. Let the tubes stand for 5 min.

4. Centrifuge all serum-containing tubes and controls for 10 min at 800 to 1000 × g, and transfer the supernates to the labeled 12 × 75 mm cuvets.

5. Set the wavelength to 540 nm, and adjust the spectrophotometer to 100% transmittance with the blank. Measure the absorbance, A, of the standard, patients' specimens, and controls at 540 nm.

Calculations

Calculate the concentration of salicylate (as salicylic acid) as follows:

$(A_{specimen}/A_{standard}) \times 200$ = salicylate, mg/L.

Convert to mmol/L by dividing this result by 138 mg/mmol.

Quality Control of Procedure

The range of linearity of the method should be checked when the method is first used and then periodically as described below. One need not prepare a standard curve for each set of specimens, provided the quality-control results remain within acceptable limits and the spectrophotometer is stable. Prepare a new standard curve if any of the following occur: use of new standard or new reagent, adjustment or repair of the instrument, use of a different instrument, transport of the instrument, unusual or possibly erroneous results on patients' specimens or controls, or six months since the last standard curve was prepared. To prepare a standard curve, dilute 1, 2, 5, 10, and 25 mL of the stock salicylate standard to 100 mL with water to prepare working standards of 20, 40, 100, 200, and 500 mg/L.

Results and Discussion

Interferences. Drugs, anticoagulants, bilirubin, and hemoglobin were evaluated for possible interference with the method. Aqueous solutions of the potential interferents were added to a pool of human serum that had been fortified with sodium salicylate. We analyzed these and the aqueous solutions of the potential interferents themselves as described above; the results are summarized in Table 1.

In contrast to another report (9), we found that acetoacetate and oxalate do not interfere at the concentrations given in Table 1. Hemoglobin does not interfere, because it is precipitated by the Trinder reagent. A highly icteric serum yielded a very faintly yellow solution after addition of the Trinder reagent; the bilirubin probably precipitates with its carrier protein, albumin.

Table 1. Interferences with the Trinder Method for Salicylate

Substance and concn added to serum, mg/L		Salicylate concn, mg/L		
		Before substance added	After substance added[a]	Apparent change
Acetoacetic acid, Li salt	17	183	176	−7
	100[b]	0	9	9
Ascorbic acid	167	183	176	−7
	1000[b]	0	0	0
Bilirubin	55	164	166	2
	104	110	117	7
	152	55	56	1
	201	0	10	10
Citric acid	167	183	177	−6
	1000[b]	0	0	0
Na$_2$EDTA	167	183	175	−8
	1000[b]	0	2	2
Hemoglobin	5700	209	212	3
Heparin	20 000[c]	219	213	−6
L-DOPA	167	183	194	9
	1000[b]	0	231	231
Methyl-DOPA	83	183	188	5
	500[b]	0	96	96
Oxalic acid, Na$_2$ salt	167	183	178	−5
	1000[b]	0	0	0
Tetracycline	83	183	193	10
	1000[b]	0	230	230
Tobramycin	27	183	178	−5
	160[b]	0	0	0

[a]Apparent salicylate concentration. [b]Aqueous solution of substance. [c]Units/L.

Both L-DOPA and methyl-DOPA gave falsely increased results, with the interference from L-DOPA being more serious. Serum fortified with L-DOPA at 167 mg/L slowly darkened on standing and became opaque after standing overnight.

L-DOPA, methyl-DOPA, and tetracycline appear to give a nonspecific increase in absorbance, reacting with the Trinder reagent to give an unknown but interfering chromophore (see Table 1). With L-DOPA, the reaction with the reagent continues for hours, darkening the solution. At the usual therapeutic concentrations of tetracycline (1 to 10 mg/L), however, tetracycline does not interfere (1, p 285).

Linearity. Serial dilutions of the stock standard were prepared to obtain solutions ranging from 15.63 to 1000 mg of salicylate (expressed as salicylic acid) per liter. Each dilution and the stock standard were analyzed in duplicate by the above method. The results are shown in Figure 1. Results by the method vary linearly with concentration, well into the toxic region of >500 mg/L, to at least 1000 mg/L, and are usable with negligible error to 2000 mg/L.

Analytical recovery studies. Inter-related specimens were prepared to check the recovery of salicylate from specimens having the same matrix. We supplemented 25 mL of a serum pool having an original concentration of 41 mg of salicylate per liter with either 4 mL of the 2000 mg/L stock salicylate standard or 4 mL of water. These two pools were mixed in various ratios to give the expected concentrations of salicylate shown in Table 2, and were analyzed by the above method. The measured concentrations of salicylate agreed well with the calculated (expected) concentrations, except for the lowest-concentration specimens, which gave higher results than expected. The Evaluator's findings agreed with ours. We conclude that the method has adequate accuracy and recovers the expected concentrations of salicylate when there is no change in the matrix. The higher-than-expected recovery at 100 mg/L is inconsequential, this concentration being in the lower analgesic-therapeutic range.

Table 2. Analytical Recovery Studies

Salicylate concn, mg/L		
Expected	Measured	% recovery[a]
Submitters		
311	308	99
256	254	99
201	206	102
146	159	109
90	97	108
35	43	123
Evaluator		
200	206	103
600	594	99
1000	970	97

[a](Expected/measured) × 100.

Reproducibility. We analyzed two commercially available controls, both within-day and between-day. Our precision results and those of the Evaluator are shown in Table 3. We conclude the method has satisfactory precision when performed as described.

Color stability. The formation of the iron-salicylate complex is essentially instantaneous. To determine the stability of the color, we analyzed the abnormal Dade control, measuring its absorbance over 2.5 h. We checked the 100% transmittance setting with the blank before each reading. The absorbance readings as a percent of the first reading (and time of the reading) were: 100% (start), 100.8% (35 min), 100.4% (60 min), 100.2% (90 min), 101.5% (130 min), and 101.2% (150 min). Therefore, measuring the absorbance of a sample within 2 h of running the reaction should produce acceptable results.

Comments. Because the absorbance at 540 nm is a linear function of salicylate concentration to well over 1000 mg/L, the method is usable from the low therapeutic to the distinctly toxic range. For emergency toxicology, the method gives acceptable results to 2000 mg/L, slightly underestimating values above about 1500 mg/L. We also studied the results for the method with 0.5 mL of serum

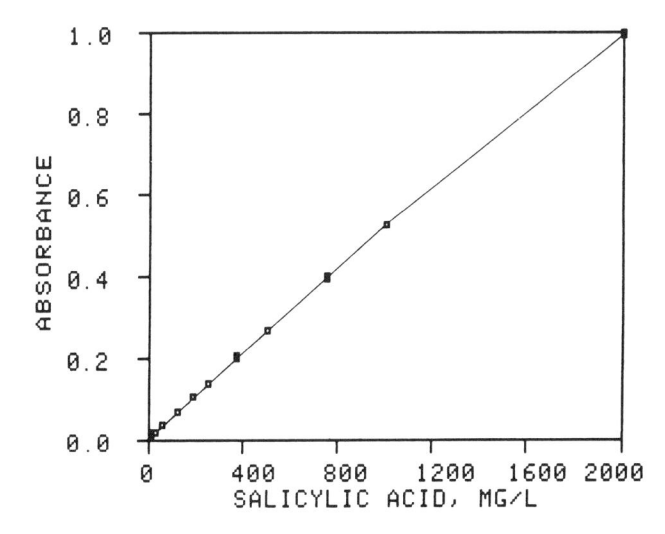

Fig. 1. Calibration plot for Trinder method
Note some loss of linearity between 1000 and 2000 mg/L. The equation for the line is $y = (4.99 \times 10^{-4}) x + (9.558 \times 10^{-3})$; $r = 0.9996$

Table 3. Precision Studies

Control	n	Salicylate, mg/L Mean	SD	CV,%
Within-day: Submitters				
Normal[a]	20	110	4.0	3.6
Abnormal[a]	20	276	7.2	2.6
Between-day: Submitters				
Normal[a]	44	108	2.8	2.6
Abnormal[a]	80	276	5.9	2.1
Within-day: Evaluator				
	20[b]	44	2.0	4.5
	20[b]	489	7.0	1.4
Between-day: Evaluator				
	16[b]	49	3.0	6.1
	16[b]	482	10	2.1

[a]Normal-XLS and Abnormal-XLS; American Dade, Miami, FL 33152.
[b]TDM Level I and TDM Level II; Ortho Diagnostic Systems Inc., Westwood, MA 02090.

and 2.5 mL of Trinder reagent. This procedure was more precise (CVs for control sera were about one-half of those cited above) and more accurate in the low-concentration range, but this approach requires more specimen volume, and the calibration curve is linear to only 400 mg/L.

The Trinder reaction is relatively free of interferences, with the exceptions described in Table 1. Others have described interferences from *p*-aminobenzoic acid and furosemide, which retard the clearance of salicylate, and from corticosteroids, which tend to reduce serum salicylate by an in vivo effect. Glucose, phenols, and urea have no effect on the procedure (9).

References

1. Bochner F, Carruthers G, Kampmann J, et al. Acetylsalicylic acid. In *Handbook of Clinical Pharmacology*, Little, Brown and Co., Boston, MA, 1966, pp 90-92.
2. Amrein PC, Ellman L, Harris WH. Aspirin-induced prolongation of bleeding time and perioperative blood loss. *J Am Med Assoc* **245**, 1825-1828 (1981).
3. Smith FA. Therapeutic drug monitoring of theophylline, salicylates, and acetaminophen. *Clin Lab Med* **1**, 567-573 (1981).
4. Boston Collaborative Drug Surveillance Group. Regular aspirin intake and acute myocardial infarction. *Br Med J* i, 440-443 (1974).
5. Hill JB. Salicylate intoxication. *N Engl J Med* **288**, 1110-1113 (1973).
6. Levy G. Clinical pharmacokinetics of aspirin. *Pediatrics* **62** (Suppl), 867-872 (1978).
7. Done AK. Significance of measurements of salicylate in blood in cases of acute ingestion. *Pediatrics* **26**, 800-807 (1960).
8. Trinder P. Rapid determination of salicylate in biological materials. *Biochem J* **57**, 301-303 (1954).
9. Garrett PE. Salicylate. In *Selected Methods for the Small Clinical Chemistry Laboratory*, WR Faulkner, S Meites, Eds., AACC, Washington, DC, 1982, pp 337-340.
10. Levy G, Tsuchiya T, Amsel LP. Limited capacity for salicyl phenolic glucuronide formation and its effect on the kinetics of salicylate elimination in man. *Clin Pharmacol Ther* **13**, 258-268 (1972).

Tricyclic Antidepressants by Gas-Liquid Chromatography with a Nitrogen-Sensitive Detector (Provisional)[1]

Submitters: Jerry L. McHan and Gerald Long, *Pathologists' Service, P. A. Atlanta, GA 30302*

Introduction

Numerous techniques have been reported for estimating concentrations of tricyclic antidepressant drugs in plasma, as comprehensively reviewed by Scoggins et al. (*1*) and Van Brunt (*2*). The only techniques currently practical for most laboratories are those involving chromatography. Both gas-liquid chromatography (GC) and "high-performance" liquid chromatography are used for monitoring tricyclics. In the methods described here a simple and rapid column-extraction method precedes a GC technique in which the same internal standard is used for determining all of the following tricyclic antidepressants: amitriptyline and nortriptyline, imipramine and desipramine, doxepin and desmethyldoxepin.

Principle

The columns for prechromatographic extraction contain a modified form of diatomaceous earth that adsorbs aqueous samples and distributes them over a larger surface area. Solvent added to the columns comes in contact with the film of aqueous sample on the diatomaceous earth, extracts the drugs, and is then collected with the analyte and removed from the sample by evaporation. The principles of liquid-liquid extraction apply to this type extraction—i.e., the ionic state of the drug of interest will affect the efficiency of the extraction. For example, tricyclics (weak bases) that do not ionize at a high pH (e.g., in the K_2CO_3 buffer) will be extracted into the organic phase (hexane) if the columns are adjusted to pH 10 before the solvent is added. The organic phase is filtered through the column and is cleaned up by the unsaturated part of the column matrix. It is important not to saturate the column with serum or aqueous buffer because the clean-up area will be overfilled and the serum components will leak through the bottom of the column into the collection tubes.

The drugs are chromatographed on an OV-17-type column and detected with a nitrogen-phosphorus detector. With cyproheptadine as the internal standard (*3*), amitriptyline, doxepin, imipramine, and their secondary amine metabolites can all be quantified.

Materials and Methods

Equipment and Supplies

"Clin Elut" columns (cat. no. 1003; Analytichem International, Harbor City, CA; also available through other suppliers).

A Model 5840A gas chromatograph with nitrogen-phosphorus detector (Hewlett Packard Corp., Palo Alto, CA) equipped with a 1.83 m × 2 mm (i.d.) glass column, packed with 3% SP-2250 (Supelco Inc., Bellefonte, PA 16823). The temperatures of the injection port, column oven, and detector are 250 °C, 265 °C, and 350 °C, respectively. The flow rate of the carrier gas, helium, is 30 mL/min.

Reagents

1. *Extraction buffer: potassium carbonate/diethylamine.* Dissolve 250 g of anhydrous K_2CO_3 in water; dilute to 1000 mL and add 4 mL of diethylamine. Solution stable for three months when stored in a brown glass bottle at room temperature.

2. *Hexane.* Use HPLC-grade only.

3. *Bovine serum albumin solution.* Weigh 9 g of NaCl, 5 g of sodium azide, and 50 g of bovine serum albumin (Cohn Fraction V, cat. no. A-9647 or A-8022; Sigma Chemical Co., St. Louis, MO) into a 1-L flask. Add 800 mL of distilled water and stir for approximately 1 h. Filter to remove any particulate matter, using a large Whatman filter paper. Dilute to 1 L with distilled water. Solution stable for one month stored at 4-7 °C.

4. *Benzene/diethylamine.* Add 20 µL of diethylamine to 20 mL of pesticide-grade benzene. Make fresh solutions daily.

Standards

1. *Stock internal standard.* Dissolve 48 mg of cyproheptadine (Periactin; Merck Sharp and Dohme, West Point, PA) in 50 mL of isopropanol containing 0.1 mL of concentrated NH_4OH. Dilute to 100 mL and shake vigorously for 10 to 15 min to ensure a uniform final concentration, 480 mg/L. Solution stable for a year when stored in a brown glass bottle at 4-7 °C.

2. *Working internal standard.* Dilute 4 mL of cyproheptadine standard to 100 mL with isopropanol. Final concentration is 19.2 mg/L; stable for three months stored in a brown glass bottle at 4-7 °C.

3. *Stock standard of tricyclic antidepressants.* Dissolve 28 mg of amitriptyline HCl and 28 mg of nortriptyline HCl in isopropanol containing 0.1 mL of concentrated NH_4OH and dilute to 100 mL with isopropanol. Final concentration is 250 mg/L each. Similarly, prepare standards for the imipramine-desipramine pair and for

---

[1] This chapter is marked "provisional," indicating that it has not met the criteria of our reviewing process. However, the method is used daily in the Submitters' laboratory, and not only is clinically useful, but also has met standards of quality for many years.

doxepin-desmethyldoxepin. Solution stable for a year when stored in a brown glass bottle at 4-7 °C.

4. *Intermediate stock standard.* Dilute, separately, 4 mL of each stock standard to 100 mL with isopropanol. Final concentration is 10 mg/L each. Solution stable for three months when stored in a brown glass bottle at 4-7 °C.

5. *Pipetting standard.* Dilute, separately, 5 mL of intermediate stock standard to 200 mL with 50 g/L bovine serum albumin solution. Final concentration is 250 µg/L; stable for two weeks in a brown glass bottle at 4-7 °C.

Collection and Handling of Specimens

Blood samples collected either into heparinized glass syringes, or by another suitable method, should be centrifuged and the plasma separated as quickly as possible. Historically, plasticizer in the rubber stopper of some collection tubes, e.g., Vacutainer Tubes (Becton Dickinson and Co.), reduced the apparent plasma concentration of tricyclics but this is not a problem in newer tubes. However, one should be alert to the possibility of variation in results caused by changes in a manufacturer's formulation.

Procedure

1. Label 16 × 125 mm tubes for blank, standards, quality controls, and patients' samples. Place these tubes in the lower section of the column stand. Fit the upper section over the tubes and insert the Clin-Elut columns into the stand, making sure the tips of the columns extend into the tubes.

2. Add 1 mL of extraction buffer to each column.

3. Add 50 µL of cyproheptadine working internal standard to each column. Because this is a small volume, gently touch the pipet tip to the gauze on top of the column packing material.

4. Add 2 mL of bovine serum albumin solution to the blank. Add 2 mL of standards, quality controls, and patients' serum samples to the appropriate columns. Allow the columns to adsorb the samples for 3 to 5 min.

5. Add 4 mL of hexane to each column and let it filter through the column at its own pace. Wash each column with another 4 mL of hexane and let drip until completely finished.

6. Place the tubes in a 56 °C water bath and evaporate the hexane, being careful to remove the tubes once they have dried, to prevent any loss of drugs.

7. Dissolve the residue in each tube with 50 µL of benzene/diethylamine and inject 5 µL of this into the gas chromatograph. The drugs will elute according to Figure 1. Their relative retention times are given in Table 1.

Table 1. Retention Time of Tricyclics Relative to Cyproheptadine

	Relative retention time
Amitriptyline	0.58
Nortriptyline	0.66
Imipramine	0.64
Desipramine	0.73
Doxepin	0.67
Desmethyldoxepin	0.76
Cyproheptadine (internal standard)	1.0

Calculations

Divide the peak height of each drug standard by the peak height of the internal standard. Next, calculate a multiplication factor for each standard by dividing the concentration of the standard by its corresponding peak-height ratio. Average the multiplication factors and use that value (W) to calculate the drug concentrations in the

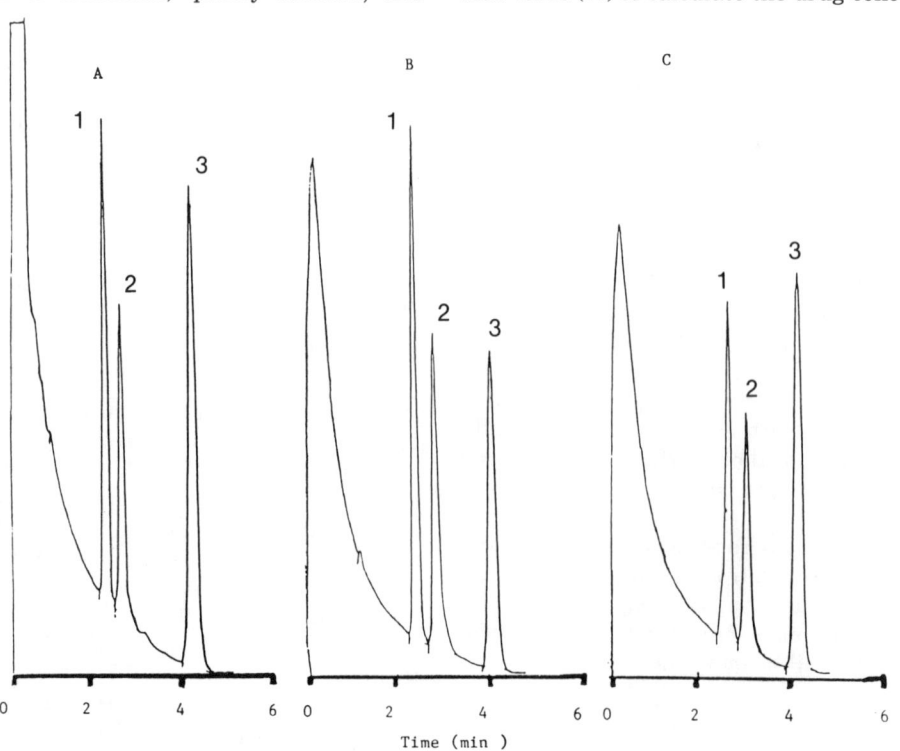

Fig. 1. Chromatograms of drug-free serum containing 250 µg/L of each pair of tricyclics: *A*, amitriptyline *(1)*, nortriptyline *(2)*, internal standard *(3)*; *B*, imipramine *(1)*, desipramine *(2)*, internal standard *(3)*; *C*, doxepin *(1)*, desmethyldoxepin *(2)*, internal standard *(3)*

Table 2. Precision of the Method

| | \multicolumn{6}{c}{Within run} | \multicolumn{6}{c}{Between run} |
	AMI	NORT	IMI	DES	DOX	NORD	AMI	NORT	IMI	DES	DOX	NORD
Target value, µg/L	125	125	125	125	125	125	125	125	125	125	125	125
SD, µg/L	7.8	9.1	4.1	8.4	7.5	10.5	6.4	10.8	7.0	8.4	4.9	10.0
CV, %	6.2	7.3	3.3	6.7	6.0	8.4	5.1	8.6	5.6	6.7	3.9	8.5
Target value, µg/L	250	250	250	250	250	250	250	250	250	250	250	250
SD, µg/L	8.0	9.8	9.3	20.3	9.3	12.5	9.3	10.3	8.0	18.5	10.8	15.0
CV, %	3.2	3.9	3.7	8.1	3.7	5.0	3.7	4.1	3.2	7.4	4.3	6.0

AMI, amitriptyline; NORT, nortriptyline; IMI, imipramine; DES, desipramine; DOX, doxepin; NORD, desmethyldoxepin. n = 20 each.

quality controls and patients' samples. To calculate these latter values, multiply the average multiplication factor, W, by the peak-height ratio of the corresponding drugs to get the concentration for each sample. To summarize:

$$W = \frac{\text{concn of standard } (\mu g/L)}{\text{peak-height ratio (drug/int. std.)}}$$

W × peak-height ratio of unknown in sample or quality control = concn, µg/L.

Discussion

Use of the column-extraction technique not only reduces the sample preparation time substantially—from 2 h to 30 min—but also improves precision of the assay, making it comparable with that of the better solvent-solvent extraction methods (2).

Table 2 summarizes the analytical precision data for the determination of these tricyclic drugs. The coefficients of variation were based on replicate determinations of sera supplemented with 125 and 250 µg/L of each pair of tricyclics.

The method is sensitive enough to detect each drug at 5 µg/L, and the range of linearity extends from 25 to 300 µg/L. Analytical recovery, based on a comparison of relative peak areas of extracted serum samples with those of nonextracted methanolic standards, was as follows (mean of n = 10 determinations each): amitriptyline, 82%; nortriptyline, 81%; imipramine, 80%; desipramine, 78%; doxepin, 77%, desmethyldoxepin, 82%.

References

1. Scoggins BA, Maguire KP, Norman TR, Burrows GD. Measurement of tricyclic antidepressants. Part I. A review of methodology. *Clin Chem* **26**, 5-17 (1980).
2. Van Brunt N. Application of new technology for the measurement of tricyclic antidepressants. *Ther Drug Monit* **5**, 11-37 (1983).
3. Nyberg G, Martensson E. Quantitative analysis of tricyclic antidepressants in serum from psychiatric patients. *J Chromatogr* **143**, 491-497 (1977).
4. Bertrand M, Dupuis C, Gagnon M, Dugal R. Nanogram-range determination of plasma imipramine by gas-liquid chromatography using a selective nitrogen/phosphorus detector. *Clin Biochem* **11**, 117-120 (1978).
5. Dawling S, Braithwaite RA. Simplified method for monitoring tricyclic antidepressant therapy using gas-liquid chromatography with nitrogen-detection. *J Chromatogr* **146**, 449-456 (1978).
6. Bailey DN, Jatlow PI. Gas-chromatographic analysis for therapeutic concentrations of amitriptyline and nortriptyline in plasma, with use of a nitrogen detector. *Clin Chem* **22**, 777-781 (1976).
7. Vasiliades J, Bush KC. Gas-liquid chromatographic determination of therapeutic and toxic levels of amitriptyline in human serum with a nitrogen-sensitive detector. *Anal Chem* **48**, 1708-1711 (1976).
8. Gifford LA, Turner P, Pare CMB. Sensitive method for the routine determination of tricyclic antidepressants in plasma using a specific nitrogen detector. *J Chromatogr* **105**, 107-113 (1975).
9. Cooper TB, Allen D, Simpson GM. A sensitive GLC method for the determination of imipramine and desmethylimipramine using a nitrogen detector. *Psychopharmacol Commun* **1**, 445-454 (1975).

Tricyclic and Tetracyclic Antidepressants by Liquid Chromatography

Submitters: E. Howard Taylor and Richard H. Gadsden, Sr., *Division of Clinical Chemistry, Department of Laboratory Medicine, Medical University of South Carolina, Charleston, SC 29425*

Evaluator: John Wojcieszyn, *International Clinical Laboratories, Nashville, TN 37202*

Introduction

Tricyclic and tetracyclic antidepressant drugs in serum are monitored to evaluate several possibilities: patients' compliance; toxicity, especially in patients with concurrent cardiac, renal, or liver disease; adequacy of clinical response to a certain dose or maximization of therapeutic benefit; and potential overdose (1,2). Currently available methods for this monitoring include: radioimmunoassay, homogeneous enzyme immunoassay (EMIT™), gas chromatography, and "high-performance" liquid chromatography (HPLC). Scoggins et al. (3) present an excellent review of methodology.

Immunologic methods for measuring these drugs lack specificity because the antisera cross react with both tertiary and secondary tricyclic amines (4). The gas-chromatographic methods attempted (5) involve use of nitrogen/phosphorus detectors, electron-capture detectors, or mass spectrometry, which makes these procedures unattractive for routine clinical laboratory use. HPLC offers an inexpensive and practical alternative. Extraction of the drugs from alkaline plasma with an organic solvent or by a column extraction procedure is followed by either reversed-phase, ion-pair partition, or adsorption chromatography with ultraviolet detection. These HPLC methods require 10 to 20 min to run, making them suitable for routine laboratory procedures. Tricyclics are well separated by reversed-phase HPLC (6, 7); however, in one reversed-phase method presented (8), some compounds (29 of about 200 tested) may interfere. Although many of the interfering drugs are unlikely to be prescribed with tricyclics, an ion-pairing reversed-phase method (9) or a CN-bonded-phase method (10), both of which show fewer interferences, may be preferred. Use of a silica column has also been described to encounter few interferences (11).

Numerous procedures for solvent extractions have been described (3). However, the use of a column for extracting the drugs from plasma eliminates the need for centrifugation and for transferring organic solvents. Column extraction also reportedly reduces the adsorption of tricyclics onto glass (10), thus increasing the absolute recovery by as much as fourfold, in an automated column-extraction procedure (12). We have modified this method (12) slightly and present here three possible extraction methods for tricyclic and tetracyclic drugs and their determination by HPLC.

Principle

Tricyclic and tetracyclic antidepressants are extracted from plasma by one of these methods: (a) manual solvent extraction with hexane; (b) manual column extraction on a C_{18} resin; or (c) an automated column extraction on a styrene divinylbenzene resin. The organic extract is then dried and reconstituted with 100 µL of mobile phase; 30 µL of this is injected into an HPLC containing a CN-bonded-phase column. The drugs are detected by their absorbance at 254 nm. Concentrations are calculated by comparing peak-area ratios of unknowns with those of standards.

Materials and Methods

Standards and Reagents

1. *Standards*: Prepare stock solutions of the following drugs, 100 mg/L of methanol: amitriptyline (Merck Sharp and Dohme, West Point, PA 19486), imipramine (Ciba Pharmaceutical Co., Summit, NJ 07901), doxepin, and desmethyldoxepin (Pfizer Labs., New York, NY 10017).

For the stock solutions of nortriptyline, desipramine, trimipramine, maprotiline, and protriptyline solutions, we used tablets of Aventyl (Eli Lilly and Co., Indianapolis, IN 46202), Norpramin (Merrell National Labs., Cincinnati, OH 45215), Surmontil (Ives Labs Inc., New York, NY 10017), Ludiomil (Ciba Phamaceutical Co.), and Vivactil (Merck Sharp and Dohme), respectively.

Evaluator's note: The stock standard solutions were stable for at least three months.

Prepare working standards by diluting stock solutions to 4 mg/L with de-ionized water. Standards are stable for three months when stored at 4 °C. The serum-based standard (400 µg/L) used in the assay is prepared by adding 100 µL of working standard to 900 µL of drug-free serum.

2. *Internal standard*: Dilute the stock protriptyline solution to a concentration of 10 mg/L in distilled water.

3. *Organic solvents*: Acetonitrile, chloroform, methanol, and hexane (Burdick and Jackson Labs., Muskegon, MI 49442).

4. *Sodium bicarbonate*: $NaHCO_3$, 80 g/L (0.95 mol/L) in distilled water.

5. *Mobile phase*: Prepare 500 mL of a 710 mg/L (5 mmol/L) solution of Na_2HPO_4. Adjust the pH to 7.9 with saturated NaH_2PO_4 and filter through a 0.45-µm pore-size HAWP 04700 filter (Millipore Corp., Bedford, MA 01730). Add 300 mL of methanol and 1200 mL of acetonitrile (total volume 2 L). De-gas the mobile phase by stirring and

passing nitrogen through the solution at a rate of 200 mL/min for 15 min. Keep the mobile phase capped and stirred while in use.

6. *Eluting solvents for column extraction*: For the automated extraction method use methanol/acetone/methylene chloride (5/1/15, by vol). For the manual column extraction use 770 mg (10 mmol) of ammonium acetate per liter of methanol.

7. *Control material*: We used control sera for imipramine, desipramine, amitriptyline, and nortriptyline from Utak Labs., Inc., Saugus, CA 91350.

Apparatus

HPLC system: The HPLC system consists of a Model M6000A solvent delivery system, a Model 440 ultraviolet detector, a WISP 710B auto injector, a Data Module 730, and a system controller 720 (all from Waters Associates, Milford, MA 01756). Either of two types of cyanopropyl (CN) columns can be used: a 10 cm × 8 mm Radial-Pak CN cartridge that fits into a Z module™ radial compression separation system, or a 30 cm × 4 mm stainless steel column packed with a CN silane-coated silica resin (all from Waters Associates). Both types of columns contain 10-μm-diameter particles of packing material but are used with different flow rates, owing to the lesser back pressure with the radial compression column. The flow rate of mobile phase through the radial compression column is 4.0 mL/min, through the stainless steel column 2.5 mL/min. The eluted drugs are detected by measuring the absorbance at 254 nm with 0.005 A full-scale deflection. The chart speed is 0.5 cm/min and the run time is 16 min.

Automated column extraction: For automated extraction, we have successfully used a Prep I automated sample processor and disposable resin cartridges packed with Type W styrene divinylbenzene copolymer (E.I. du Pont de Nemours, Clinical Systems Division, Wilmington, DE 19898). Twelve samples can be processed at once.

Manual column extraction: For the manual column extraction method we used a Vac-Elut system and disposable columns (Bond-Elut) packed with a C_{18} bonded phase (Analytichem International, Inc., Harbor City, CA 90710). With this system one can prepare 10 samples at once.

Collection and Handling of Specimens

Collect blood into glass tubes containing either sodium citrate or potassium oxalate/sodium fluoride. We used blue-stopper or grey-stopper Vacutainer Tubes (Becton, Dickinson and Co., Rutherford, NJ 07070). In response to early reports of decreased plasma values because of the plasticizer tris(2-butoxyethyl) phosphate in the rubber stopper (*3*), Vacutainer Tubes manufactured since 1978 contain a new formulation that does not affect the concentrations of tricyclics (*10*). Centrifuge the whole-blood sample (3000 × g for 5 min) as soon as possible, at least within 24 h. The plasma may then be stored at 4 °C for several days before analysis without observed decreases in drug concentrations.

Procedures

Preparation of buffered sample: To 1 mL of patient's plasma, serum-based standard, or control serum, add 200 μL of the $NaHCO_3$ buffer. Extract the drugs from this buffered sample by one of the following methods.

Automated extraction: Load the buffered sample onto the Type W extraction column. Fill the Prep I solvent reservoir I with 20 mL of distilled water and solvent reservoir II with 21 mL of the methanol/acetone/methylene chloride eluting solvent. Set the Prep I for program no. 15 according to the manufacturer's instructions, with the evaporation temperature at 68 °C. The Prep I is a reversible centrifuge that allows the sample to pass through a preparatory column. The resin is flushed to remove any unadsorbed solute, and this wash is collected in a waste cup. The rotor then reverses direction and dispenses organic solvent, which elutes the adsorbed analytes from the column. The extracts are collected in aluminum cups and automatically dried. Reconstitute the dried extract in the aluminum recovery cup with 100 μL of mobile phase and vortex-mix for 15 s. Inject 30 μL of this into the HPLC.

Manual column extraction: Insert a Bond-Elut column into each holder of the Vac-Elut system. Aspirate through each column 2 mL of methanol, twice, followed by 2 mL of distilled water, twice. Turn off the vacuum source and add all of the buffered sample to each column. Reduce the pressure again and wash each column with three 1-mL aliquots of distilled water, followed by three 1-mL aliquots of methanol. Under normal pressure, elute the analytes with 200 μL of the methanolic ammonium acetate. Wait about a minute to allow the eluate to drain, then reduce the pressure again to remove the rest of the eluate. Repeat this elution step two additional times, then evaporate the combined eluate under nitrogen at 60 °C. Reconstitute the dried extract with 100 μL of mobile phase, vortex-mix for 15 s, and inject 30 μL into the HPLC.

Manual solvent extraction: Add 5 mL of hexane to the buffered sample. Vortex-mix for 30 s, then centrifuge (3000 × g) for 5 min. Transfer the clear hexane (top layer) to another tube and evaporate it at 60 °C under a stream of nitrogen. Reconstitute the dried extract with 100 μL of mobile phase, vortex-mix for 15 s, and inject 30 μL into the HPLC.

Calculations

Concn of sample, μg/L = (AR sample/AR stand) × concn of standard (400 μg/L), where AR = area ratio: peak area of tricyclic of interest/peak area of internal standard (whether in the sample or the standard solution).

These calculations represent the concentration of the tricyclic base. If the HCl forms are used, one must account for this difference in mass—e.g., 277.39 vs 313.84 for amitriptyline base and amitriptyline·HCl, respectively. If one has prepared standards from amitriptyline·HCl, the concentration of the standard (amitriptyline base in the above calculations) then becomes 400 × 277.39/313.84 = 353.54 μg/L.

Discussion

Figure 1 shows the resolution of seven tricyclic antidepressants by this HPLC method. Doxepin was not included in this composite standard because it co-elutes with amitriptyline. The tetracyclic, maprotiline, is not resolved from protriptyline. Drug-free serum does not show any peaks, and there is no difference in background from any of the three different methods of extraction (Figure 2). A plot of peak-area ratio (analyte/internal standard) against concentration is linear to at least 1000 μg/L for each analyte (*12*).

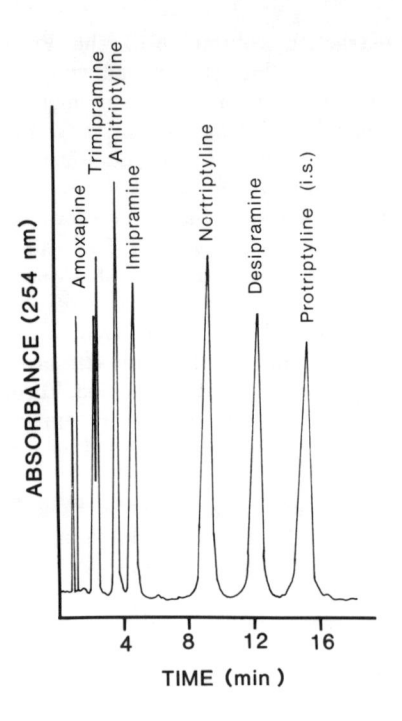

Fig. 1. **Chromatographic separation of seven tricyclic antidepressants by HPLC**

Amounts injected were: amoxapine (45 ng), trimipramine (60 ng), amitriptyline (120 ng), imipramine (120 ng), nortriptyline (240 ng), desipramine (240 ng), and protriptyline (900 ng)

For the secondary amines (desipramine and nortriptyline) the detection limit in serum is 10 µg/L for the manual solvent extraction and 5 µg/L for the column-extraction methods. The detection limits for the tertiary amines (doxepin, amitriptyline, and imipramine) are even lower, about 3 µg/L. All of these far exceed the lower end of the therapeutic range (50 µg/L). Absolute recovery ranges from 20 to 44% with the manual solvent extraction and from 72 to 97% with the automated column extraction; analytical recoveries vary from 92 to 107%. Within-run CV (n = 12, with 100 µg/L added to serum) averages 10.1 and 6.0% for the manual solvent extraction and the automated column extraction, respectively. Run-to-run CVs (n = 10, with 100 µg/L added to serum) averaged 10.7 and 6.7% for the manual solvent extraction and the automated column extraction, respectively.

All three methods of extraction are satisfactory for routine measurement of tricyclic antidepressants. The automated sample method allows increased sensitivity because of greater absolute recovery and takes less time for sample preparation: for 12 samples, 40 min vs 90 min by the manual solvent extraction.

We examined possible interference by some other drugs. The first seven drugs listed in Table 1 co-elute near the void volume. The following interferences are possible and should be considered in reporting results for co-administered medications: trifluoperazine with amoxapine and trimipramine; thioridazine and procainamide with doxepin and amitriptyline; and disopyramide and desmethyldoxepin with nortriptyline. Also, as stated earlier, doxepin and amitriptyline co-elute. In clinical situations where maprotiline or protriptyline is used, a different internal standard, desmethyldoxepin, must be used.

New or soon to be released antidepressant drugs such as aprazolam (Xanax; Upjohn, Kalamazoo, MI 49001), trazadone (Desyrel; Mead Johnson, Evansville, IN 47721), mianserin (Organon, West Orange, NJ 07052), nomifensine (Merital; Hoechst-Roussel, Somerville, NJ 08876), and bupropion (Wellbutin; Burroughs Wellcome, Research Triangle, NC 27709) should also be examined under these chromatographic conditions.

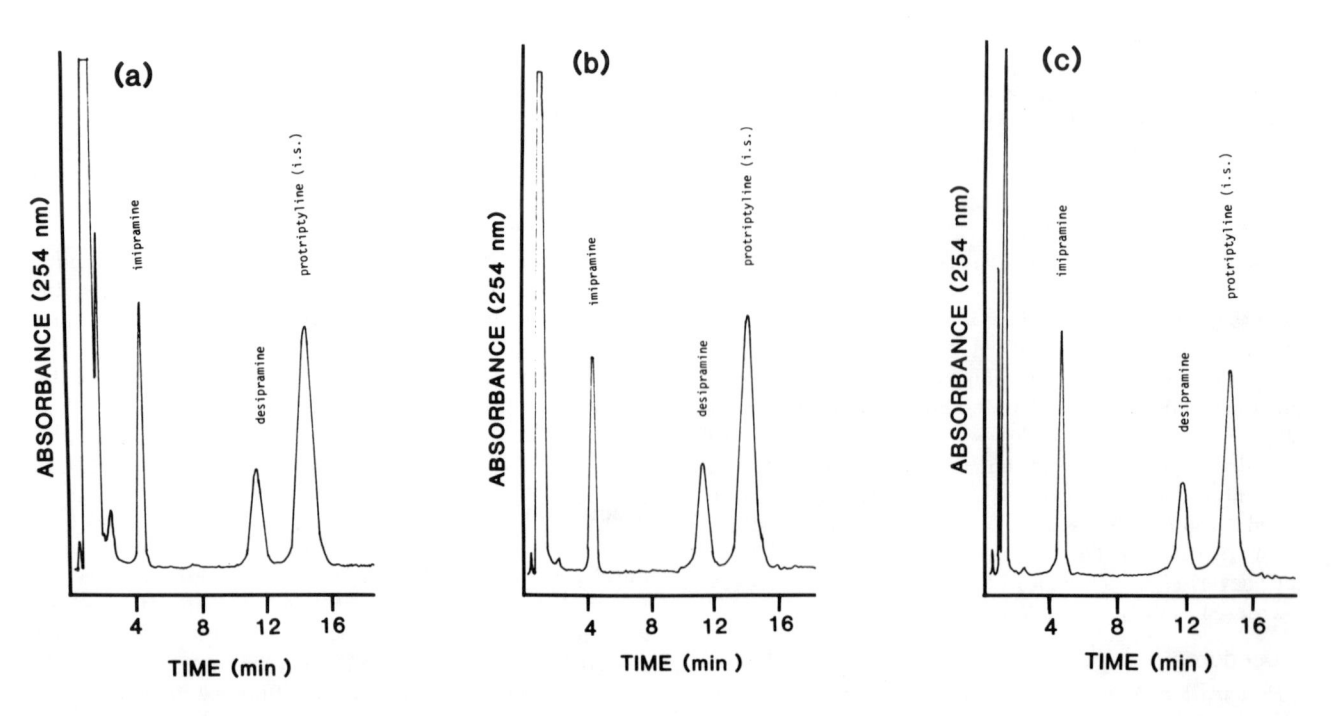

Fig. 2. Chromatogram of a serum-based standard containing 400 µg/L each of imipramine and desipramine after treatment by each of three extraction procedures: (a) automated column extraction, (b) manual column extraction, and (c) manual solvent extraction with hexane containing 20 mL of n-butanol per liter

For details of each method, see text. i.s., internal standard

Table 1. Column Capacity Factors (K′)[a] of Common Drugs

Drug	K′	Drug	K′
Caffeine	0.90	Doxepin	6.34
Theophylline	0.91	Amitriptyline	6.66
Salicylate	0.94	Thioridazine	6.88
Chlordiazepoxide	2.32	Propranolol	6.92
Methaqualone	2.32	Propoxyphene	7.30
Diazepam	2.40	Imipramine	8.06
Acetaminophen	2.45	Desmethyldoxepin	11.30
Amoxapine	4.23	Nortriptyline	17.50
Trifluoperazine	4.96	Disopyramide	17.52
Trimipramine	5.04	Desipramine	19.17
Chlorpromazine	5.30	Maprotiline	24.80
Procainamide	6.34	Protriptyline	25.70

[a] K′ = $(T_d - T_o)/T_o$, where T_d = absolute retention time of drug, and T_o = absolute retention time of void volume.

Evaluator's Comments

Linearity/precision study. As recorded with a strip-chart recorder, the standard curves for the tricyclics amitriptyline, nortriptyline, imipramine, and desipramine showed linearity to 1000 μg/L. For doxepine and desmethyldoxepin linearity extended only to 400 μg/L. The demonstrated precision was as summarized in Table 2.

Accuracy study. I used the manual extraction method of Hebb et al. (*J Anal Tox* 6: 206-208, 1982) and an "in-house" HPLC method, and monitored the column eluate at 215 nm. Drug-supplemented sera (150 μg of the tricyclics listed per liter) were prepared and analyzed by both methods, with the following results (means of 10 determinations each):

Tricyclic	Evaluator's "in-house" method	Submitters' method
Amitriptyline	180.0	146.1
Imipramine	180.0	170.3
Nortriptyline	165.1	138.7
Desipramine	181.0	142.0

To the prepared sera (n = 10), I added an additional 400 μg of the tricyclics per liter and analyzed them by the Submitters' method. Analytical recoveries were as follows: amitriptyline, 86.9-116.1%; imipramine, 86.3-115.4%; nortriptyline, 80.0-103.1%; desipramine, 86.9-119.7%; desmethyldoxepin, 80.2-109.2%.

References

1. Scoggins BA, Maguire KP, Norman TR, Burrows GP. Measurement of tricyclic antidepressants, II. Applications of methodology. *Clin Chem* **26**, 805-815 (1980).
2. Van Brunt N. The clinical utility of tricyclic antidepressant blood levels: A review of the literature. *Ther Drug Monit* **5**, 1-10 (1983).
3. Scoggins BA, Maguire KP, Norman TR, Burrows GD. Measurement of tricyclic antidepressants, I. A review of methodology. *Clin Chem* **26**, 5-17 (1980).
4. Maguire KP, Burrows GD, Norman TR, Scoggins BA. Evaluation of a kit for measuring tricyclic antidepressants. *Clin Chem* **26**, 529 (1980). Letter.
5. Van Brunt N. Application of new technology for the measurement of tricyclic antidepressants using capillary gas

Table 2. Results of the Evaluator's Precision Studies with This Method

	Within-run precision				Between-day precision			
	Concn, μg/L				Concn, μg/L			
Level	Mean	SD	CV, %	n	Mean	SD	CV, %	n
Amitriptyline								
Low	50.9	5.4	10.7	7	56.2	10.6	18.8	10
Med.	107.0	35.5	30.1	13	146.1	30.1	20.6	34
High	417.7	27.6	6.6	9	389.5	59.7	15.3	18
Desipramine								
Low	53.4	8.1	15.1	10	50.2	8.4	16.8	
Med.	139.0	23.7	17.0	14	142.8	3.0	2.1	34
High	400.0	10.2	2.5	9	398.8	27.7	6.9	18
Desmethyldoxepin								
Low	48.8	5.5	11.2	9	53.7	7.7	14.3	
High	395.6	17.5	4.4	9	390.0	39.6	10.1	17
Imipramine								
Low	50.4	4.5	9.0	9	54.3	8.6	15.8	12
Med.	155.8	22.2	14.3	13	170.3	28.3	16.6	34
High	399.4	21.6	5.4	9	390.0	39.6	10.1	17
Nortriptyline								
Low	51.4	2.3	4.6	10	54.2	5.9	10.9	11
Med.	140.1	21.7	15.5	13	138.7	1.6	1.1	34
High	401.0	10.7	2.7	9	390.9	28.1	7.2	18

chromatography with a fused silica DB5 column and nitrogen phosphorus detection. *Ther Drug Monit* **5**, 11-37 (1983).

6. Johnson SM, Chan C, Cheng S, et al. Isocratic high-performance liquid chromatographic method for the determination of tricyclic antidepressants and metabolites in plasma. *J Pharm Sci* **71**, 1027-1030 (1982).

7. Kabra PM, Mar NA, Marton CJ. Simultaneous liquid chromatographic analysis of amitriptyline, nortriptyline, imipramine, desipramine, doxepin, and nordoxepin. *Clin Chim Acta* **111**, 123-132 (1981).

8. Bannister SJ, Van der Wal SJ, Dolan JW, Snyder LR. Liquid chromatographic analysis for common tricyclic antidepressant drugs and their metabolites in serum or plasma with the Technicon "Fast-LC" system. *Clin Chem* **27**, 849-855 (1981).

9. Proelss HF, Lohman HJ, Miles DG. High performance liquid chromatographic simultaneous determination of commonly used tricyclic antidepressants. *Clin Chem* **24**, 1948-53 (1978).

10. Thoma JJ, Bondo PB, Kozak CM. Tricyclic antidepressants in serum by a Clin-Elut™ column extraction and high pressure liquid chromatographic analysis. *Ther Drug Monit* **1**, 335-338 (1979).

11. Sonsalla PK, Jennison TA, Finkle BS. Quantitative liquid chromatographic technique for the simultaneous assay of tricyclic antidepressant drugs in plasma or serum. *Clin Chem* **28**, 457-461 (1982).

12. Koteel P, Mullins RE, Gadsden RH. Sample preparation and liquid chromatographic analysis for tricyclic antidepressants in serum. *Clin Chem* **28**, 462-466 (1982).

Index

Acetaminophen 23, 24, 33-39, 99
Acetone 40-43, 64, 85, 88
Alcohols 7, 40-43, 85; *see also* Ethanol
American Association for Clinical Chemistry 11
Amphetamines 13, 16, 18-20
Anticonvulsant drug control material 7
Antidepressant drugs, *see* Tetracyclic, Tricyclic
Arsenic 44-46
Atomic absorption spectrophotometry 75-78, 79-81

Barbiturates 11, 13, 18-20, 23, 47-50
Basic drugs (in urine) 26-29
Benzodiazepines 2, 19
Blind specimens 5, 9, 11
Blood gas 54
Bromide 51-52

Calibration standards 7
Cannabinoids 2
Carbon monoxide/carboxyhemoglobin 2, 53-56
Centers for Disease Control (CDC) 1, 11, 77
Cerebrospinal fluid 2, 4, 41, 51, 90
Chain of custody/evidence 1
Chlorinated hydrocarbons 31
Cocaine 13, 16, 19, 20, 24
Codeine 13, 16, 19, 20, 24, 27
Collection of specimens 2, 4, 78
College of American Pathologists (CAP) 1, 11
Cyanide 2, 57-62

Detection limits 11
Drugs, *see* Screening *and specific drug of interest*

Enzymic analyses 63-65, 86-87
Error, allowable limit of 9
Ethanol 2, 40-43, 63-65, 85-88
Ethanolic intoxication 1, 85
Ethchlorvynol 16, 24, 66-67
Ethylene glycol 64, 69-71, 85, 87, 88

Ferrozine 72
Forensic pathologists 4
"FPN" test 30
Fujawara reaction 31

Gas chromatography, head-space method 31, 40-43, 65
Gas-liquid chromatography (GLC) 22-25, 69-71, 93-95
Gastric contents, assays with 1, 2, 4, 15, 19, 20, 29, 31, 45, 57, 58, 66, 82
Glutethimide 13, 16, 18, 20-21, 24-25

Hair 45
Handling of specimens 2, 4, 7, 12
Head-space gas chromatography, *see* Gas chromatography
Hydrocarbons, chlorinated 31

Internal standard 6
Informed consent 1
Iron 72-74
Isopropanol 40-43, 64, 85, 87, 88

Lead 2, 11, 75-78
  Poisoning, risk classification 77
Levey-Jennings control chart 8-9
Liquid chromatography (HPLC) 33-34, 96-99

Mass spectroscopy 9
Matrix 5, 7
Medico-legal implications 1, 2, 5
Meprobamate 13, 16, 19-21, 23, 25
Mercury 79-81
Methanol 40-43, 64, 85, 87, 88
Methaqualone 16, 20, 23, 25, 82-84, 99
Microdiffusion 53, 57-62
Morphine 1, 13, 16, 19, 20, 25
Multiple drugs, screening/assay 4, 13-25

Nicotine 7, 20, 25, 27

Osmometry, freezing-point depression 40, 85-88

Phencyclidine (PCP) 17, 19, 23, 26
Phenobarbital 6, 18, 23, 49
Phenothiazines 19, 30
Pills and capsules, assay of 15, 19, 28
Plasma specimens 2, 7, 22, 41, 57, 58, 63, 90, 93, 97
Preservation of specimens 4
Proficiency testing 9, 11, 77

Quality assurance 5-12
Quality-control materials 5-9, 11, 14, 87
Quality-control statistics 9

Reference publications 2, 6

Salicylate 7, 17, 21, 50, 89-92, 99
Saliva 2, 4
Sample handling 2, 4, 7, 12
Screening for drugs 9, 13-31, 66-67
  Basic drugs in urine 26-29
  By gas-liquid chromatography 22-25
  By thin-layer chromatography 10, 13-21
  Chlorinated hydrocarbons 31
  Phenothiazines 30
Sensitivity 20-21
Serum specimens 2, 7, 22, 33, 37-38, 41, 51, 57, 58, 63, 66, 77-78, 82, 85-86, 90, 97
Shewhart chart 8-9
Specificity 5
Spectrophotometric assays 47, 51, 57, 66, 71, 82, 89

TBP (tetrabromophenolphthalein ethyl ester) 26-29
Tetracyclic antidepressants 96-99
Therapeutic Drug Monitoring (TDM) 5, 6, 9, 11
Thin-layer chromatography (TLC) 5, 9-11, 13-21
Thiocyanate 57-62
Tricyclic antidepressants 13, 19, 20, 28-29, 93-99
Trinder method 89

Urine specimens 1, 2, 5, 7, 9, 11, 15-21, 26-29, 30, 31, 45, 57, 58, 63, 66, 79, 86

Venipuncture 1, 2
Vitreous Fluid 41, 63
"Volatiles" 2, 40, 85; *see also* Ethanol

Whole-blood specimens 2, 42-43, 45, 54, 57, 58, 63, 75, 86